D0969773

THERAPY TECHNIQUES
FOR CLEFT PALATE SPEECH
AND RELATED DISORDERS

THERAPY TECHNIQUES FOR CLEFT PALATE SPEECH AND RELATED DISORDERS

Karen J. Golding-Kushner, Ph.D.

Assistant Professor
Department of Special Education and Individualized Services
Speech Pathology Program
Kean University
Union, New Jersey
And
Private Practice,
East Brunswick, New Jersey

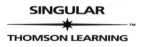

SINGULAR

™

THOMSON LEARNING

Australia   Canada   Mexico   Singapore   Spain   United Kingdom   United States

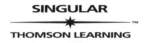

SINGULAR

™

THOMSON LEARNING

Therapy Techniques For Cleft Palate Speech and Related Disorders
by Karen J. Golding-Kushner, Ph.D.

Business Unit Director:
William Brottmiller

Acquisitions Editor:
Marie Linvill

Editorial Assistant:
Cara Jenkins

Executive Marketing Manager:
Dawn Gerrain

Channel Manager:
Kathryn Bamberger

Executive Production Editor:
Barb Bullock

Production Editor:
Brad Bielawski

COPYRIGHT © 2001 by Singular, an imprint of Delmar, a division of Thomson Learning, Inc. Thomson Learning™ is a trademark used herein under license

Printed in Canada
5 XXX 06 05 04 03

For more information contact Singular,
401 West "A" Street, Suite 325, San Diego, CA 92101-7904
Or find us on the World Wide Web at
http://www.singpub.com

ALL RIGHTS RESERVED. No part of this work covered by the copyright here-on may be reproduced or used in any form or by any means—graphic, electronic, or mechanical, including photocopying, recording, taping, Web distribution or information storage and retrieval systems—without written permission of the publisher.

For permission to use material from this text or product, contact us by
Tel (800) 730-2214
Fax (800) 730-2215
www.thomsonrights.com

Library of Congress Cataloging-in-Publication Data Available upon request

NOTICE TO THE READER

Publisher does not warrant or guarantee any of the products described herein or perform any independent analysis in connection with any of the product information contained herein. Publisher does not assume, and expressly disclaims, any obligation to obtain and include information other than that provided to it by the manufacturer.

The reader is expressly warned to consider and adopt all safety precautions that might be indicated by the activities herein and to avoid all potential hazards. By following the instructions contained herein, the reader willingly assumes all risks in connection with such instructions.

The Publisher makes no representation or warranties of any kind, including but not limited to, the warranties of fitness for particular purpose or merchantability, nor are any such representations implied with respect to the material set forth herein, and the publisher takes no responsibility with respect to such material. The publisher shall not be liable for any special, consequential, or exemplary damages resulting, in whole or part, from the readers' use of, or reliance upon, this material.

Contents

Foreword

This volume represents a unique project in a number of ways. First and foremost, it is a book devoted solely to the clinical management of a specific speech disorder that, although fairly common, is also often misunderstood, misdiagnosed, and mistreated. Speech disorders associated with cleft palate and velopharyngeal insufficiency (VPI) have traditionally been managed in hospital settings, and as such, a relatively small number of speech pathologists have had the opportunity to see many cases or study the problem. However, problems associated with VPI are common enough so that most clinicians in public schools and other clinical settings encounter patients occasionally. When they do, although they are mandated to treat these cases, they are often left wondering what therapeutic techniques to apply. This book represents tried and true procedures that are based on thousands of hours of clinical experience as applied by some of the leading clinicians in the world who have devoted their careers to the management of cleft palate, VPI, and related disorders. There is a second unique aspect of this text.

Although written by a single author, Karen J. Golding-Kushner, Ph.D., this text was conceived and gestated by a panel of scientists and clinicians who have devoted their careers to studying the speech problems associated with VPI. The technique for establishing the content of this book is one that has been tried once before successfully. In 1990, an International Working Group was assembled to write a position statement on the standardization of diagnostic procedures for VPI, a project that was also written and reported by the author of this text and published in *The Cleft Palate-Craniofacial Journal* (Golding-Kushner, et al. 1990). Our current project brought together a panel of clinical experts to develop a focus for the content and techniques described in this text. We met at Upstate Medical University, Syracuse, NY in January, 2000, working nearly nonstop until we had met our objective. In addition to the author, the participants included (in alphabetical order): Linda D'Antonio, Ph.D. (Loma Linda University and Children's Hospital, Loma Linda, CA); John Riski, Ph.D. (Children's Healthcare of Atlanta, Atlanta, GA); Robert J. Shprintzen, Ph.D. (Upstate Medical University, Syracuse, NY), Mary Anne Witzel, Ph.D., University of Toronto, Ontario, Canada, and Antonio Ysunza, M.D., Sc.D. (Hospital Gea Gonzales, Mexico City). Each of the participants in this consensus group has extensive clinical experience with cleft palate and VPI and all of us have large numbers of publications in the scientific literature spanning many years. All of us are clinicians who have, for at least 20 years and in some instances 30 years, worked in hospital settings in some of the largest and most active craniofacial and cleft palate centers in the world. Our cumulative experience spans many thousands of patients and all of us have been teachers of speech pathology students, medical and dental residents, and clinicians. It was the intent of this project to offer a volume that would be written in the same manner that we instruct our own students.

Two grants were awarded to allow this meeting to take place. One grant came from the publisher, Singular Publishing Group, who enthusiastically supported this project from its inception. The second grant came from The Velo-Cardio-Facial Syndrome Educational Foundation, Inc. for reasons that will be discussed below. Our working group met, talked, argued, and agreed on the material so ably integrated by Dr. Golding-Kushner. More than a consensus opinion, this volume represents a concerted effort to make an emphatic statement to clinicians about what works and what does not.

The third unique aspect of this text is the existence of a grass roots effort by parents of a special group of patients to see this project come to fruition. Velo-cardio-facial syndrome (VCFS) is one of the most common multiple anomaly syndromes in humans and one of the most frequent clinical findings in the syndrome is speech characterized by VPI, hypernasality, and abnormal articulation. This group of patients has always presented a special problem to clinicians because of the severity of the problem and the frequent failure of speech therapy. The techniques described in this book have been particularly effective in children with VCFS. The Velo-Cardio-Facial Syndrome Educational Foundation, Inc. is an organization whose purpose is to educate both professionals and the public about VCFS and its treatment. At its annual meeting in Milwaukee in 1999, the membership and Board of Directors of the Foundation agreed to support this project so that the therapy procedures proven to be so successful in children with VCFS could finally reach print. The Foundation with several thousand members around the world maintains a web site at *www.vcfsef.org*.

It is important for us to acknowledge the contributions of several other individuals who participated in this process. Participating in the January meeting was Natalie Havkin, M.S., staff clinician at the Communication Disorder Unit, Department of Otolaryngology and Communication Science of Upstate Medical University and speech pathologist for the Center for the Diagnosis, Treatment, and Study of Velo-Cardio-Facial Syndrome. As an active clinician whose practice consists largely of children with cleft palate and/or VCFS, she served as an excellent sounding board for the group and she contributed admirably to the process. Kelvin Ringold, Administrative Assistant for the Communication Disorder Unit, made all of the necessary arrangements that managed to bring our panel together from disparate points to snowy Syracuse with amazing precision and without a flaw. Marie Linvill of the Singular Publishing Group was critical to the success of this project, being the first person to listen to the idea. She has been the project's main facilitator, allowing us to finish this text in a matter of months.

To my colleagues and dear friends Linda (D'Antonio), Jay (John Riski), Mary Anne (Witzel), and Tony (Ysunza), a very special thank you. They all took time out of their very busy schedules to participate in this project without compensation. They recognized this as important and their collegiality and friendship represents the best that professionals have to offer each other. Their cooperation shows the highest level of ethical conduct in wanting this knowledge to reach the public as a result of this project, even though any one of them could have written a book similar to this one on their own. This is a group of preeminent and superb scientists who came because they recognize that together, as one, we could make an impact that exceeded the sum of our parts.

Finally, special mention needs to be made of the author, Karen J. Golding-Kushner, Ph.D., and the invaluable task she has performed. She wrote this book within an amazingly short time facing the challenge of cohesively joining the thoughts of our esteemed panel. I have known Dr. Golding-Kushner for many years, as far back as her undergraduate studies. She was my student and my employee over the years, but now she is simply my respected colleague. Many of the techniques described in this text are her original concepts. Unlike many scientists, Dr. Golding-Kushner has been able to bridge the academic world and clinical world with alacrity. She is a superb diagnostician and therapist who has had a major impact on this field. I could think of no one better to write this text, and no one better to champion the techniques described within.

Robert J. Shprintzen, Ph.D.
Director, Communication Disorder Unit
Director, Center for the Diagnosis, Treatment, and Study of Velo-
    Cardio-Facial Syndrome
Director, Center for Genetic Communicative Disorders
Professor of Otolaryngology and Communication Science
Upstate Medical University
Syracuse, NY

Consensus Group

This text was conceived by a group of specialists known internationally for their work with individuals with cleft palate, VPI, and related disorders. This group of specialists from across North America met for several days to talk about what therapy procedures really *do* work with this often hard-to-treat group of patients. Participants were (in alphabetical order):

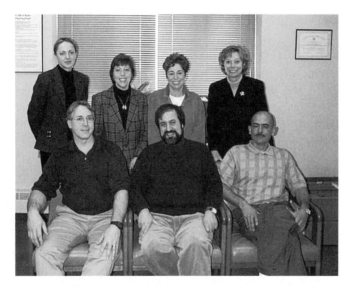

Front row left to right: Riski, Shprintzen, Ysunza
Back row left to right: Natalie Havkin, M.S. (Guest), Golding-Kushner, D'Antonio, Witzel

Linda L. D'Antonio, Ph.D., CCC-SLP
Professor, Department of Surgery
Loma Linda University and Children's Hospital
Loma Linda, CA

Karen J. Golding-Kushner, Ph.D., CCC-SLP
Assistant Professor, Department of Special Education and
    Individualized Services
Speech Pathology Program
Kean University
Union, New Jersey
Private Practice
East Brunswick, New Jersey

John E. Riski, Ph.D., CCC-SLP, FASHA
Director, Speech Pathology Laboratory
Clinical Director, Center for Craniofacial Disorders
Children's Healthcare of Atlanta
Atlanta, GA

Robert J. Shprintzen, Ph.D., CCC-SLP , FASHA
Professor and Director
Communication Disorder Unit,
Department of Otolaryngology and Communication Science
Center for the Diagnosis, Treatment, and Study of Velo-Cardio-Facial
    Syndrome
State University of New York Health Science Center at Syracuse
Upstate Medical University
Syracuse, NY

Mary Anne Witzel, Ph.D., CCC-SLP
Associate Professor, Adjunct Faculty
Department of Speech-Language Pathology
University of Toronto
Ontario, Canada

Antonio Ysunza, M.D., Sc.D.
Clinical Research Department
Hospital Gea Gonzales
Mexico D.F., Mexico

Acknowledgments

I received a phone call from Bob Shprintzen last fall asking how I felt about finally sitting down to write a book we had discussed many times over the last 23 years. It would be a book about how to do speech therapy with children who had glottal stop speech, and would include procedures I had used and talked about at conferences many times. It was not until we had talked for half an hour that he confessed having already discussed this project with both the Board of Directors of the Velo-cardio-facial Syndrome Educational Foundation and Marie Linvill at Singular Publishing Group. I was sure that the chapters I had written for other texts contained everything I had to say on the subject, but Bob, as usual, persevered. He described his vision of gathering a group of experts to form a consensus group to formulate the structure of the book and talk about our experiences with different treatment protocols and procedures. The opportunity to get together with Bob, Mary Anne, Linda, Jay, and Tony was too exciting to pass up. I agreed to write the book as my ticket to brain storm for two days with this group of internationally recognized experts that I have long held in high esteem.

To say that the two day meeting was an incredible professional experience would be an understatement. It was an honor to sit among these experts, and I am grateful to each member of the group for their insight and direction, their thoughtful comments on the manuscript as each chapter was written in the weeks and months that followed our meeting and, especially, for their confidence in my ability to write this therapy guide. I believe that the finished product truly represents the consensus on what procedures work, which ones should be avoided, and why. I hope that I have represented our collective experience adequately.

I am extremely fortunate to have had Dr. Robert J. Shprintzen as my teacher and mentor for well over twenty-five years, and I am especially proud to also call him my colleague and friend. As always, Bob was confident that I could write this book when I had doubts. I am extremely grateful for his encouragement and support at every stage of this project.

I would also like to thank the Board of Directors of the Velo-cardiofacial Syndrome Educational Foundation, Inc. for their support. Without their grant, the consensus group meeting would not have occurred and this book would probably not have been written. Thank you to

Marie Linvill, Brad Bielawski, and the staff at Singular Publishing Group. Their grant also made the consensus group meeting possible. Marie was very supportive from the project's inception. I appreciated her gentle reminders of looming deadlines that helped keep me on track and her patience with all of my questions. Brad's keen attention to detail was of great assistance.

Thank you to Dr. Ana Maria Schuhmann, Dean of The School of Education, and Dr. Elaine Fisher, Chair of the Department of Special Education and Individualized Services at Kean University. My special appreciation to the faculty of the Speech Pathology Program at Kean, Dr. Martin Shulman, Dr. Mary Jo Santo Pietro, Dr. Sheree Reese, Dr. Barbara Glazewski, Dr. Barbara Lecomte, and Professor Alan Gertner. They have welcomed me warmly and expressed their support as I worked on the final stages of this project while assuming the responsibilities of a full time faculty position.

Finally, I would like to thank my husband, Stuart, my son, Leor and my daughter, Tzipora, for their encouragement and understanding. Okay guys, Mommy can play now!

Dedication

To the children with cleft palate and VPI and their parents:
Keep your sight on the goal of normal speech.

CHAPTER

Introduction

This is a book about speech therapy for individuals with cleft palate, velopharyngeal insufficiency (VPI)[1], and their sequelae. Its purpose is to provide information that will be useful to clinicians and parents of children with "cleft palate speech." It is a "How To" book with a developmental approach, conceived because of frequent requests for information from speech-language pathologists being asked to offer therapeutic services to individuals with cleft palate at various stages of development. Types of interventions that may be provided by speech specialists treating children with cleft palate and related disorders, including feeding, early intervention, prevention, and treatment of speech disorders are described, along with recommendations about when treatment should be applied. It is also a book about how practicing speech-language pathologists (SLPs) can guide parents through the therapy process, not just to understand it, but to participate in it.

It is not within the scope of this book to review various other types of treatment, such as surgical or dental procedures. However, SLPs working with this population should be familiar with those other aspects of treatment, and many excellent books are available on those subjects (Bardach & Morris, 1990; McWilliams et al., 1990; Shprintzen & Bardach, 1990).

---

[1]It has been suggested that the terms velopharyngeal *insufficiency, inadequacy,* and *incompetency* be used to differentiate VP dysfunction of various causes. All three are abbreviated VPI and the term velopharyngeal *insufficiency* is used generically in this text.

DEBUNKING THE MYTHS

The second chapter of this book is devoted to some commonly held misconceptions about cleft palate and speech. It is hoped that by dismissing these myths, the reader will be able to focus on the many positive aspects of the prevention and treatment of speech errors associated with cleft palate.

HOW SPEECH IS PRODUCED. . . .
AND WHAT GOES WRONG

Children born with cleft palate may exhibit speech problems related to many anatomic and medical problems, such as velopharyngeal insufficiency, palatal fistulae, dental malocclusions, and chronic or fluctuating hearing loss. Children with clefts are also prone to the same phonological and developmental articulation disorders exhibited by other children. However, the focus of this book will be the special circumstances that lead to the sometimes complex communicative impairments associated with orofacial anomalies. Understanding the mechanics of speech production and the nature of speech errors provides a framework for developing appropriate treatment plans. The process of normal speech production will be reviewed in Chapter 3, and a model of what goes wrong during speech development when a baby is born with a cleft palate will be described. Speech errors associated with cleft palate and velopharyngeal insufficiency (VPI), such as nasal emission, nasal snorting, and glottal stops will be defined within that model. A classification system to assist SLPs and parents in determining if errors are developmental, obligatory, or compensatory is provided as a basis for establishing programs for the prevention of errors and treatment when they occur.

THE SLP AND INFANTS WITH CLEFT
PALATE: PREVENTION AND EARLY TREATMENT

SLPs may be asked to meet with parents of newborns to educate them about cleft palate and to provide assistance with feeding. SLPs also provide guidance regarding early speech and language development, and should monitor the emergence of vocalizations from the earliest discomfort and comfort cries and sounds, through vocalic cooing, the development of consonantal babbling, and production of the first word. Early intervention, parent counseling, feeding, early monitoring and prevention are discussed in Chapter 4.

BEYOND EARLY INTERVENTION: FROM PRESCHOOL THROUGH ADOLESCENCE

Models for service delivery for children age 3 years and older are considered in Chapter 5. Included is information about scheduling, group and individual therapy, Individualized Educational Plans (IEPs), and a discussion about the type of speech therapy that might be needed at different stages of development and medical intervention.

HOW TO CHANGE SPEECH PATTERNS

It is often assumed that speech therapy for children with clefts is difficult and that the errors are resistant to change. Many procedures have been found to work both effectively and quickly. Procedures for the elimination of maladaptive compensatory errors are described in detail in Chapter 6. Establishing use of correct production in words, sentences, and conversation is considered in Chapter 7. Chapter 8 provides information about materials and procedures that have proven to be useful in the treatment of "cleft palate speech," and Chapter 9 describes procedures that should be avoided.

VELO-CARDIO-FACIAL SYNDROME

Velo-cardio-facial syndrome (VCFS) is the most common syndrome associated with cleft palate and velopharyngeal insufficiency. It is of special importance to SLPs because communication and learning disorders are among the most frequent and perplexing features of the syndrome. VCFS and suggested treatment approaches are discussed in Chapter 10, along with other syndromes and conditions.

CHAPTER

2

Speech Therapy Won't Help .... and Other Myths

Some SLPs and parents approach the prospect of speech therapy for children with cleft palate with undue concern about the process. Unfortunately, there is a substantial amount of misinformation in the field, in part, because many training programs have not emphasized this clinical area to any significant degree. This misinformation has led to the development of a number of persisting myths about cleft palate and associated speech disorders. So, before describing the therapy process, let us dismiss some of the common myths about speech and speech therapy. Each of these topics is examined in detail in subsequent chapters of this book.

MYTH #1: YOUR CHILD WILL NEED
SPEECH THERAPY FOR MANY, MANY YEARS

One of the first things parents of children with clefts are told is, "with surgery and therapy, your child will be fine." They are often told that the therapy will be protracted, lasting for many years. However, studies indicate that at least 80% of children born with nonsyndromic cleft palate, who undergo palate repair by 18 months of age, do not require direct speech therapy at all (Hall & Golding-Kushner, 1989; Peterson- Falzone, 1990). Children who do have speech problems related to a cleft or to velopharyngeal insufficiency may need different types of speech therapy at different stages of development. These therapy cycles must be timed correctly in relation to surgical and dental intervention. Depending on the severity of the speech problem, good and efficient treatment should not last for more than one to two years and, in some cases, even shorter periods. Although speech therapy is often required, some treatment may not be appropriate until adolescence. Therefore, it is a myth that therapy lasts "forever," but it may be true that therapy will be provided in cycles.

MYTH #2: SPEECH THERAPY WILL NOT BE EFFECTIVE UNTIL AFTER PALATE SURGERY

In relation to palate repair, most professionals agree that the optimal time for complete repair of clefts of the hard and soft palate is at or before one year of age. Children who are not babbling or "trying out" speech sounds before that time may benefit from early intervention services with a focus on vocalic and nasal sounds. If palate repair is delayed for some reason, therapy should not be deferred if it is needed and oral consonants can be taught. Residual alveolar clefts may be present until bone grafting at 8 years of age or later is accomplished, and this does not affect early speech therapy.

MYTH #3: SPEECH THERAPY WILL NOT BE EFFECTIVE UNTIL AFTER PHARYNGEAL FLAP SURGERY

Not only *can* speech therapy be effective before pharyngeal flap surgery, it is recommended in certain situations. In a speaker with errors known as "cleft palate speech," elimination of glottal stops may have a favorable effect on velopharyngeal function and lead to modification of the surgical plan (Golding, 1981; Henningsson & Isberg, 1986; Golding-Kushner, 1989, 1995; Shprintzen, 1990; Ysunza, Pamplona, & Toledo, 1992). Thus, in the case of speech therapy and pharyngeal flap surgery or other pharyngoplasty, it is usually our recommendation that surgical management of VPI be delayed until after speech therapy has eliminated abnormal compensatory articulation errors.

MYTH #4: YOU CANNOT DO ANYTHING ABOUT VPI WITH SPEECH THERAPY

You can! It might just not be in the way you think. As stated above, in children who have both VPI and articulation errors, eliminating maladaptive compensations, such as glottal stops, often has a favorable influence on velopharyngeal movement (Golding, 1981; Henningsson & Isberg, 1986; Golding-Kushner, 1989, 1995; Shprintzen, 1990; Ysunza, Pamplona, & Toledo, 1992). On the other hand, in speakers with VPI and good articulation skills, this is no myth. In the absence of abnormal compensatory errors, speech therapy should not be expected to improve consistent VPI. Furthermore, oral motor therapy, massage, icing, and blowing exercises are among the many procedures that are *not* effective in changing velopharyngeal function. Using those procedures, you *cannot* do anything about VPI (Powers & Starr, 1974; Ruscello, 1982; Starr, 1990; Van Demark & Hardin, 1990).

VPI should not be confused with hypernasality. Some speakers with hypernasality have variations of VPI, such as inconsistent VP closure during speech. In such cases, a decision about whether or not speech therapy will help must be made based on the information obtained from nasopharyngoscopic or multiview videofluoroscopic examination of velopharyngeal motion of the individual during speech. These imaging tools will provide information about whether or not speech therapy should be done and, if so, what procedures to use.

MYTH #5: DISCOURAGE SPEECH UNTIL AFTER PALATE REPAIR OR YOUR CHILD WILL LEARN ERRORS

Learning to communicate through sounds, noises, and gestures is one of the most natural things a baby does. By responding to their baby's vocal attempts, parents teach their child an essential and fundamental aspect of language—that their utterances can elicit a response. If they are discouraged from these attempts, they may learn that talking is a bad thing, which may hinder their language development. Speech should not be discouraged.

MYTH #6: YOUR CHILD IS APRAXIC

"Cleft palate speech" is characterized by abnormal (maladaptive) speech errors such as glottal stops that are often produced without any lip or tongue movement. This may give the *appearance* of muscle weakness, abnormality, or incoordination. However, lack of use of the articulators should not be confused with apraxia. Patients with compensatory articulation are often erroneously described as apraxic because it *appears* that they cannot move their tongues to execute movements. In most cases, they are not apraxic and the problem is *omission* of oral speech movements, not the inability to produce them (Golding-Kushner, 1995).

MYTH #7: YOU HAVE TO BE A
SPECIALIST TO TREAT CHILDREN WITH CLEFT PALATE

You do not have to be a "specialist" in cleft palate to treat children with clefts, but you do have to be an excellent speech-language pathologist. The skills necessary to treat children with speech problems related to cleft palate include a thorough knowledge and understanding of the physiology of speech production. The SLP must understand and be able to implement traditional articulation therapy techniques addressing place, manner, and voicing of sounds and traditional behavior modification techniques. The SLP should also know how to be a "team" player. The SLP should be willing to become a part of the child's treatment "team" and work together with the other professionals involved in the child's treatment. The SLP should be willing to hear and consider recommendations of other specialists, including other speech specialists.

MYTH #8: YOU HAVE TO WAIT FOR
SEVERAL MONTHS AFTER SURGERY TO START
(RESUME) SPEECH THERAPY

Speech therapy may be scheduled as soon after surgery as the surgeon allows and the patient feels well enough to participate. This is usually about a week or two postoperatively for palate repair or pharyngoplasty.

MYTH #9: AFTER A PHARYNGEAL
FLAP YOU HAVE TO RE-LEARN SPEECH

The speech skills achieved before surgery are not mysteriously lost during the operation. If articulation is good before the surgery to correct VPI, therapy may not be needed at all after surgery.

MYTH #10: THE CHILD CAN ONLY
SAY VOWELS AND OMITS CONSONANTS

Children with "cleft palate speech" often produce glottal stops, a consonant error produced by abrupt adduction (closure) of the vocal folds. It is often mis-heard as a consonant omission. Most of the time, the initial consonant has not been omitted. Rather, a glottal stop has been substituted.

MYTH #11: BABIES AND TODDLERS WITH CLEFT PALATE NEED ORAL MOTOR THERAPY BECAUSE THEY HAVE WEAK OR LAZY MUSCLES . . . . OR CHILDREN WITH "CLEFT PALATE SPEECH" SHOULD DO EXERCISE TO MAKE THE PALATE, TONGUE, AND LIPS STRONGER

A repaired cleft of the lip or palate does not signal the presence of weakness in the muscles, nor does the presence of compensatory speech errors. Children with clefts and "cleft palate speech" who omit lip and tongue movement from their speech production are not "lazy" and do not have "lazy muscles." Rather, they have substituted use of different muscles to produce the sounds in a different and abnormal way. Lack of muscle movement in this case results from an error in learning, not from laziness. Palatal "exercise" does not improve palate function or articulation (Powers & Starr, 1974; Ruscello, 1982; Starr, 1990; Van Demark & Hardin, 1990).

MYTH #12: MY CHILD'S SPEECH IS NOT IMPROVING BECAUSE HE IS LAZY

In most instances, if speech is not improving, it is an indication that the goals, procedures, or schedule for treatment are not optimal. It is the SLP's obligation to be sure that the treatment goals and procedures are appropriate, and that therapy is frequent and intensive. It is also the SLP's responsibility to use motivating, age appropriate materials. Parents or caregivers should be expected to supervise frequent, brief practice daily.

MYTH #13: YOUR BABY WILL HAVE FEEDING PROBLEMS

Children born with cleft palate, even complete bilateral cleft lip and palate, can bottle-feed normally. Minor adjustments may be necessary in the positioning of the baby and the bottle, in the size and type of nipple opening, and in the frequency of burping. In most cases, feeding appliances and special bottles or other equipment are not needed. Persistent difficulty with feeding may indicate the presence of other problems, such as neurological, airway, or respiratory compromise.

MYTH #14: BABIES WHO HAVE FEEDING PROBLEMS GO ON TO DEVELOP SPEECH PROBLEMS

There is no clear evidence that feeding problems cause speech problems, or that infants with feeding problems grow up to be children with speech problems. Speaking and eating occur in the pharynx, which is a shared space, and both are functions that are secondary to breathing. The interrelationship among the three functions—respiration, feeding, and speech—is complex, and problems in more than one area should not be assumed to be causative.

MYTH #15: MOST CHILDREN WITH CLEFT PALATE HAVE SIGNIFICANTLY DELAYED LANGUAGE

Children with nonsyndromic cleft lip and palate may be more likely to have language delays or disorders than their noncleft peers. However, there is wide variability in the type and severity of language impairment reported for children with clefts, and many children with cleft lip and palate enjoy normal language development. Speech pathologists must sometimes be creative in the assessment of expressive language skills of children with "cleft palate speech," to differentiate between an articulation disorder and a true impairment of expressive language.

On the other hand, children with isolated cleft palate are more likely to have a multiple anomaly syndrome than children with cleft lip with or without cleft palate. Children with syndromic cleft palate are, as a group, more likely to have receptive and expressive language delays and disorders than children with nonsyndromic clefts and must be considered at high risk. It should be understood that it is not the cleft that causes the language impairment. Rather, the cleft and the language impairment are likely to have a common cause, or pathogenesis. For example, children with velo-cardio-facial syndrome are likely to have both a cleft palate *and* a significant language delay, both of which are caused by a genetic deletion. Conversely, some syndromes, such as van der Woude syndrome, are *not* associated with an increased risk of language delay. Accurate diagnosis is essential in order to identify the children at high risk.

MYTH #16: VPI CAUSES LANGUAGE DELAY/DISORDERS

VPI is a physiological activity affecting one specific aspect of speech production. VPI causes hypernasality and nasal escape of air. It may predispose some individuals to learn compensatory misarticulations, such as glottal stops. However, it does not cause language delays, which are related to cognitive activity, not physiological activity.

MYTH #17: YOUR CHILD IS TOO YOUNG FOR SPEECH THERAPY . . . . OR IF SPEECH THERAPY IS NOT WORKING, THE CHILD IS NOT READY

No child is too *young* for therapy, but therapy must be geared to the age and developmental level of the child. Infants and toddlers are among the best responders to an informal-looking but carefully planned and executed play approach to sound stimulation. This is because they are less set in their abnormal patterns of sound production and can learn new patterns without having strongly established abnormal patterns to eliminate. Speech therapy for the youngest of infants may take the form of training parents to provide excellent modeling and stimulation. Treatment may become more structured and formal as the child's ability to understand and handle increasingly direct therapy increases, usually around age 3 or 4 years.

MYTH #18: ALL SPEECH THERAPY IS THE SAME

Unfortunately, not all speech therapy is the same. Just because a child has had two or more years of treatment with little or no progress, one should not conclude that the situation is hopeless. If the goals of treatment are appropriate but there has been minimal improvement, it should be assumed that the child needs a different therapy approach or a more frequent therapy schedule.

MYTH #19: GIVE HIM SOME TIME AND HE WILL OUTGROW IT

"Cleft palate speech" is not a developmental disorder. That is, children who have developed a pattern of "cleft palate speech" do not outgrow their articulation disorder (Phillips, 1990). Furthermore, when glottal patterns have been established, time acts as an enemy, strengthening the habit patterns that must be broken to learn to produce correct speech patterns.

MYTH #20: SLPS NEED EQUIPMENT
THAT IS SPECIALIZED AND EXPENSIVE TO WORK
WITH CHILDREN WITH CLEFTS;
IT WILL BREAK THE BUDGET

Fancy and expensive equipment is not necessary. Materials that are needed are routinely found in a SLP's office and include a mirror, tongue depressors, tape recorder, picture cards, and age-appropriate motivational toys and games.

CHAPTER

3

How Speech Is Produced
.... and What Goes Wrong

Children born with cleft palate may exhibit speech problems related to a variety of anatomic and medical problems, such as malocclusions and hearing loss. They may also develop the same phonological and developmental articulation disorders exhibited by children without cleft palate. By far, the speech problems that seem to cause the greatest difficulty to speech pathologists are those related to velopharyngeal insufficiency (VPI) and palatal fistulae. In order to understand these errors, it is necessary to understand the mechanics of normal speech production and what may go wrong when there is a cleft palate.

THE SPEECH MECHANISM: A SYSTEM OF VALVES

The vocal tract can be thought of as a system of valves (Figure 3–1), modifying the airstream that originates in the lungs. Characteristics of voice are produced by the respiratory system (intensity or loudness) and larynx (fundamental frequency or pitch). We generally conceptualize the vocal tract as a tone modifier. That is, we think of the vocal tract's role in imposing resonance characteristics on the speech signal after the voice characteristics have been imposed. However, the role of the vocal tract in articulation is often overlooked. There are three primary regions of constriction in the system through which air pressure

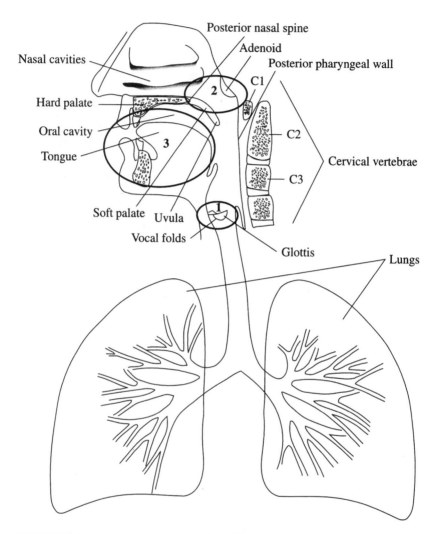

FIGURE 3–1. The vocal tract may be thought of as a system of valves, with three major regions in which modification of the airstream occurs from the time it leaves the lungs until it leaves the mouth or nose. **Valve 1:** Glottis, at the laryngeal level. **Valve 2:** Velopharyngeal region. **Valve 3:** Oral region, controlled by movement of the lips and/or tongue (tip or dorsum) and jaw. Reprinted with permission from Golding-Kushner, K. J. (1997). Cleft lip and palate, craniofacial anomalies and velopharyngeal insufficiency. In C. Ferrand, & R. Bloom (Eds.), *Introduction to neurogenic and organic disorders of communication: Current scope of practice* (pp. 193–228). Boston: Allyn & Bacon.

and airflow are modified. The inferior-most region is the laryngeal valve with primary activity at the level of the glottis. This is the valve closest to the lungs, the source of the outgoing air stream. Abduction and adduction of the vocal folds results in variations in size of the glottis which controls the laryngeal valve. The base of the tongue has attachments in the laryngeal region and has an articulatory valving function in some languages other than English. In English, phonemic lingual activity occurs in the oral region and will be discussed later.

Moving up the vocal tract, the next major region of constriction and air flow modification is the velopharyngeal (VP) area, which acts to couple or separate the nasopharynx from the oropharynx. Note that the valves are described as "regions" rather than as "points" of constriction. Velopharyngeal closure does not occur on a two-dimensional plane. VP closure has height, width, and depth. It occurs over time and space. The VP valve is controlled by elevation/retraction of the velum, anterior displacement of the posterior pharyngeal wall, which may be generalized, or localized as a Passavant's ridge, and medial (inward) movement of the lateral pharyngeal walls. Velopharyngeal closure occurs when these structures meet each other and prevent escape of air into the nasal cavity, which is a branch of the vocal tract.

The third major area of constriction along the vocal tract is the oral "valve." Airflow is controlled at the oral valve by movement of the tongue, mandible, and lips in relation to each other and to the dentition. Airflow here is controlled in various ways. Air may be permitted to flow without obstruction (as in vowels, semivowels), it may be restricted (fricative), or stopped (plosives).

Warren (1986) suggested that this system of valves is pressure-driven. That is, he believes that the system's function is based on a system in which every attempt is made to regulate pressure within the vocal tract. In this model, loss of pressure in one part of the vocal tract (that is, VPI) leads to an increase in pressure in another part of the vocal tract (at the glottis, resulting in a glottal stop). Studies of the relationship between glottal stop articulation and velopharyngeal movement support this view (Henningsson & Isberg, 1986; Hoch et al., 1986; Shprintzen, 1990; Ysunza et al., 1992; Golding-Kushner, 1989, 1995). In these studies, children with cleft palate and VPI who produced glottal stops were examined using multiview videofluoroscopy and/or nasopharyngoscopy. They were found to have poor or absent lateral pharyngeal wall motion. Following a brief period of speech therapy in which correct placement and air control for oral consonant production were taught, they were reexamined. Most of the children still had VPI but with significantly improved lateral pharyngeal wall motion (Figures 3–2 and 3–3). This could be explained following Warren's model.

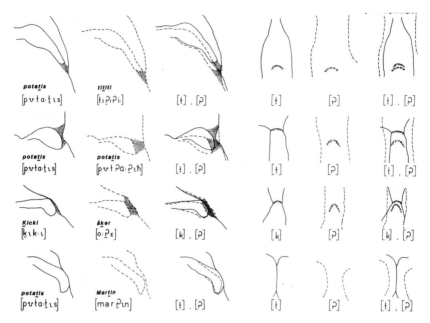

FIGURE 3–2. Tracings of velopharyngeal movements from cineradiographic frames in lateral and frontal views for oral and glottal stops. Shadowed areas indicate pharyngeal flap position. Superimposition of tracings for oral (continuous lines) and glottal articulation (dashed line) shows impairment of velopharyngeal movements for glottal articulation. Reprinted with permission from Henningsson, G. E., & Isberg A. M. (1986). Velopharyngeal movements in patients alternating between oral and glottal articulation: a clinical and cineradiographical study. *Cleft Palate Journal, 23,* 1–9.

In the presence of a loss of pressure at the VP valve (valve 2), an attempt is made to stop the airflow at an inferior (posterior) location, the glottis (valve 1), which is closer to the source of the air flow. Once that constriction is made, there is no need to constrict the air at the oral valve (valve 3), so those movements (lip, tongue) are omitted. In addition, general motion along the walls of the pharynx is decreased because of the change in rate and pressure of flow out the glottis. Furthermore, when the speakers were taught to use valve 3 (oral) correctly and to stop overuse of valve 1 (glottal), valve 2, although still deficient in most cases did, in fact, show increased motion. Clearly, learning plays a major role in the development and maintenance of compensatory speech errors.

In order to maintain the vocal fold vibration that results in production of voiced sounds, air pressure below the vocal folds (subglottal pressure) must exceed pressure above the vocal folds (Borden & Harris,

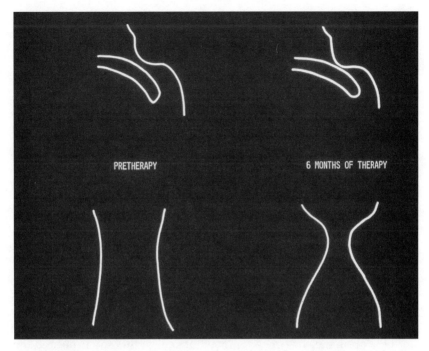

FIGURE 3–3. Tracings of lateral view videofluoroscopy (top) and frontal view videofluoroscopy during production of glottal stops prior to speech therapy, and after 6 months of articulation therapy during correct production of oral stops.

1980). Therefore, coordination of velopharyngeal and vocal fold motion plays a role in the ability to maintain voicing, in addition to adjusting the pressure and volume of the vocal tract. This may explain why many individuals with VPI and glottal stops have more difficulty producing voiced consonants than voiceless consonants, and children receiving speech therapy to correct glottal stop errors tend to have more difficulty establishing production of voiced plosives than their voiceless cognates. As will be discussed in detail later, this is one reason that, in most instances, voiceless plosives and fricatives should be introduced in speech therapy before their voiced cognates.

CLASSIFICATION OF ERRORS

Speech errors may be developmental, phonological, obligatory, or compensatory. Compensatory errors may be functional (useful) or maladaptive. Correct classification of errors is essential in order to determine treatment goals and the sequence of application of different treatment modalities.

Developmental Articulation Errors

Developmental errors are speech mistakes in which sounds are produced in a way that is normal at an earlier stage of development. Developmental errors may be substitutions, distortions, or omissions. Examples are substitution of w/r ("wabbit" for "rabbit"), and interdental lisps. This class of errors is unrelated to any structural abnormality, and should be treated in the same way as it would be in a child without a cleft or VPI. Developmental errors do not have an interrelationship with VPI. Surgical and dental treatment are inappropriate for correcting developmental errors, but may influence decisions regarding the timing of treatment for specific sounds. For example, many second and third grade children are on the caseloads of school-based SLPs to correct interdental lisps. It is developmentally appropriate to correct an interdental lisp at that age. However, if a child is receiving orthodontic treatment and wearing a maxillary expansion appliance that makes correct tongue placement difficult, therapy for sibilants should be deferred until the appliance has been removed. If speech therapy is needed for other sounds, it may proceed. In other words, even when errors are developmental in nature, the timing of speech therapy for those errors may be affected by surgical and/or dental treatment.

Phonological Errors

Phonological errors are linguistically, not phonetically based, and reflect a problem at a higher order organizational level than the phonetic errors most often associated with cleft palate. Phonological theory pertains to metalinguistic or psychological constructs and not to the physiology of speech (McWilliams, Morris, & Shelton, 1990). Children with cleft palate may have phonological errors in the sound system, just as they may have developmental errors. Phonological errors include consonant harmony, in which the speaker changes one consonant in a word to be the same as another, such as "mammer" in place of "hammer." Some reports have suggested that phonological disorders are common in children with cleft palate (Powers, 1990; Chapman, 1993; Pamplona & Ysunza, 1999a). There are some reports suggesting that the phonetic errors associated with cleft palate become incorporated into the child's rule system for sounds and, in this way, evolve into phonological disorders (Chapman, 1993; Pamplona & Ysunza, 1999a). This could be one explanation of why compensatory articulation does not correct itself when VPI and cleft palate are eliminated. It is more likely that the errors do not self correct because they are learned and integrated into the individual's speech production pattern. It is essential to maintain sight of the distinction between errors with a physiological origin (compensatory errors) and errors without an apparent physiological base, such as final consonant deletion. Clearly, nonphysiologically based phonological errors are not related to the cleft and should be considered independently.

It is essential to examine the phonetic patterns of a child's speech closely before making assumptions about phonology. This is crucial for selecting the appropriate treatment procedure. A common trap into which SLPs fall is to categorize glottal stop errors incorrectly. When a child produces glottal stop substitutions for oral consonants, the SLP may erroneously conclude that the child has a "phonological process" of "glottal replacement." This suggests that the "decision" to produce a glottal stop, albeit on a subconscious level, was made at a linguistic level, in the same way that one "decides" to sequence words in a particular order in a sentence. However, the substitution of glottal stops is a physiological error, a change made in the *motor* plan of speech. That is, it is a change in the execution of a motor act, not a change in the cognitive plan. It is a change made in order to maintain air pressure in the vocal tract and to create an acoustic event before the loss of air through a leak in the palate or VP region. The physiologically based error is likely to have been reinforced, therefore maintained and repeated, but it is not a linguistic change. As we will discuss later, this is the reason that phonological analysis and phonologically based therapy approaches are usually inappropriate with this population.

CLEFT PALATE SPEECH

"Cleft palate speech" refers to speech characteristics that are specifically associated with cleft palate and VPI and usually includes hypernasality, errors that are obligatory with VPI, such as nasal emission and weak consonants, and compensatory articulation.

Hypernasality is *not* an articulation error. It is excessive *nasal resonance* during production of vowels often associated with, but not the same as, nasal escape of air. It is usually caused by velopharyngeal insufficiency, but may also be related to the presence of a large oronasal fistula. Fistulae may cause hypernasality directly because of the anterior communication between the oral and nasal cavities. Fistulae also may cause hypernasality indirectly because the presence of a fistula may result in diminished velopharyngeal motion (Figure 3–4) (Isberg & Henningsson, 1987).

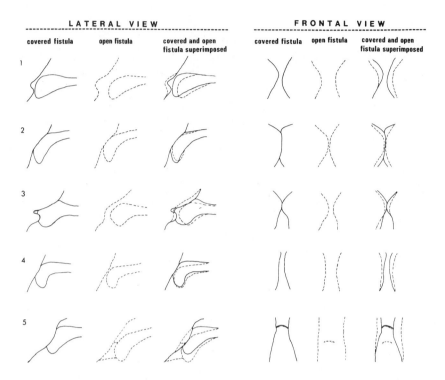

FIGURE 3–4. Tracings of velopharyngeal movements from cineradiographic frames in lateral and frontal projections during anterior articulation of pressure consonants with the fistulas covered and open, respectively. Shadowed areas represent pharyngeal flap. Superimposition of tracings for speech with covered fistulas (continuous line) and for speech with open fistulas (dashed line) shows improvement of the velopharyngeal movements during speech with the fistulas covered. Reprinted with permission from Isberg, A. M., & Henningsson, G. E. (1987). Influence of palatal fistulas on velopharyngeal movements: A cineradiographic study. *Plastic and Reconstructive Surgery, 79:*525–530.

Of the remaining characteristics of "cleft palate speech," some are obligatory, the others are learned.

Obligatory Articulation Errors

Obligatory errors are speech mistakes that are a direct consequence of an anatomic or physiological defect, and do not respond to speech therapy. They spontaneously correct when the cause of the error is corrected (Philips & Kent, 1984; Golding-Kushner, 1991, 1995). Obligatory errors include nasal emission, nasal turbulence, reduced intraoral pres-

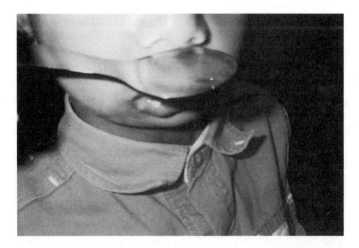

FIGURE 3–5. A small mirror held beneath the nostrils can be used to detect nasal emission during speech. Note fogging of the mirror when emission occurs.

sure resulting in weak oral consonants, and certain articulation distortions related to palatal fistulae and malocclusion.

Nasal emission is the **passive** escape of air into the nasal cavity and out the nose. Nasal emission may be silent or audible, and is most apparent during production of high-pressure consonants. Silent nasal emission may be detected by holding a small mirror or stethoscope below the nostrils (Figure 3–5). Audible nasal emission sounds like bursts of air or a steady stream of air during speech. Nasal emission is obligatory in the presence of VPI. If nasal emission is not detected in a speaker with VPI, it is because of some other nasal obstruction. When the cause of the nasal emission, whether it be VPI or a palatal fistula, is no longer present, nasal escape does not occur.

Nasal turbulence is nasal emission that passes an obstruction such as a deviated septum or congestion, and is noisy, like the rustling of leaves. It is sometimes called nasal rustle. Nasal turbulence usually occurs in bursts associated with production of pressure consonants (stops, fricatives, and affricates).

Reduced intraoral pressure results in the production of weak oral consonants. In order to produce pressure consonants, including plosives and fricatives, air pressure is built up in the mouth behind the point of constriction, or place of articulation. When air is able to escape posterior to that place, because of VPI or a fistula, intraoral pressure is reduced. This, in turn, causes the production of weak consonants. These consonants sound significantly better when the nostrils are occluded. This is because the sounds are being produced correctly but, because of a slow loss of air pressure into the nasal cavity, there is less oral air pressure to create the intended sound. Reduced intraoral pressure is a phenomenon that is detected during production of pressure consonants (stop plosives, fricatives, and affricates). It is not as noticeable during production of low-pressure sounds such as vowels and semivowels, and does not apply to nasal consonants. It is similar to the loss of efficiency of a tire on a car that has lower pressure because of a slow leak of air through an unpatched hole. The tire works, but not as efficiently as with full pressure. *Weak pressure consonants* are produced when there is insufficient intraoral pressure to create the acoustic event normally associated with consonant production. It results partially from the passive nasal emission that occurs in VPI or a large anterior fistula, and sometimes from the speaker's deliberate attempt to reduce nasal emission by talking more softly, or by using "light" articulatory contacts.

Malocclusions and other deviations in dental structure may also cause obligatory speech errors. For example, a child with an unrepaired alveolar cleft and missing teeth in the line of the cleft may use correct tongue placement and produce an oral air stream. However, because of the large interdental space, an *oral* sibilant distortion may be unavoidable (*obligatory*).

Obligatory errors do not only result from anatomic deviations. If a child is wearing certain maxillary appliances, he or she may find it impossible to achieve correct tongue placement for /s/ because of the physical interference of the orthodontic appliance (Figure 3–6). In this case, the sibilant distortion is obligatory, and therapy should be deferred until the appliance has been removed. On the other hand, if a lisp was corrected prior to insertion of the appliance, the appliance may cause a temporary obligatory distortion of the corrected speech pattern that generally returns to normal spontaneously when the appliance is removed. However, SLPs should avoid the tendency to attribute all speech errors to previously existing or remaining deviations in anatomy, and assume that errors are obligatory.

By definition, obligatory errors cannot be corrected without resolution of the underlying anatomic deviation, and therapy to correct these patterns is contraindicated. Speech therapy for obligatory errors, in addition to frustrating the child, family, and SLP, is a waste of time, energy, and financial resources.

Compensatory Errors

There are two types of compensatory errors, those that are useful and those that are not. The useful compensations may be referred to as

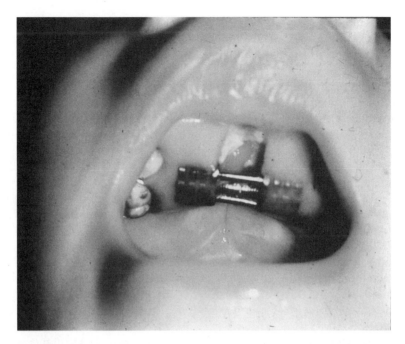

FIGURE 3–6. This maxillary expander is an example of an orthodontic appliance that may prevent the speaker from establishing correct tongue-tip placement for anterior sounds, often resulting in an obligatory sibilant distortion. Reprinted with permission from Shprintzen, R. J., & Vardach, J. (Eds.) (1995). *Cleft palate speech management: A multidisciplinary approach* (p. 323). St. Louis, MO: Mosby.

"compensatory adaptations" (Golding-Kushner, 1995). The others are usually referred to by the generic term, "compensatory errors."

Compensatory Adaptations

Compensatory adaptations include errors which are the speaker's closest possible approximation to a sound in the presence of an anatomic deviation (Golding-Kushner, 1995). Some are produced by several speakers with the same anatomic deviation, and some are unique, representing creative ways in which an individual approximates a sound. What these errors have in common is that they sound close to or exactly like the target sound, although they look incorrect. Examples of compensatory adaptations are articulatory inversions and changes in choice of articulators.

An *articulatory inversion* may be produced if a speaker has a very severe Class III malocclusion, making it impossible to achieve correct labiodental placement for /f, v/. The speaker may compensate for this by creating these sounds using the upper lip and mandibular teeth, instead of the maxillary teeth and lower lip, resulting in an "upside down" or inverted /f, v/. This usually sounds correct but looks incorrect.

Sometimes the speaker chooses *different articulators* to produce a sound. For example, an extruded or severely protruding premaxilla may interfere with lip closure and make it impossible to achieve bilabial closure for /m, p, b/. The speaker may substitute labiodental stops for /p, b/ and a labiodental nasal for /m/. The speaker typically neglects the upper lip. This may be misinterpreted as upper lip weakness, rather than upper lip disuse. The speaker should still be able to achieve lip rounding for vowels and /w/, and if he or she does not, it should not be dismissed as an adaptation. Rather, it should be considered an avoidable error and corrected in speech therapy.

Occasionally, a lip repair is very poor and results in a significant anatomic lip deficiency. This might also result in labiodental production of bilabial sounds. In this situation, the change in place of articulation would be a successful compensatory adaptation (Figure 3–7). Fortunately, this extremely negative surgical outcome does not occur frequently.

Compensatory adaptations may or may not resolve spontaneously when the anatomic deviation is corrected, but may be a logical and appropriate compensation until correct placement is possible. In fact, in some cases, speech intelligibility may be improved by teaching these compensations until physical management occurs. Unlike obligatory errors, compensatory adaptations may not spontaneously correct after the anatomic deviation is corrected, and additional speech therapy

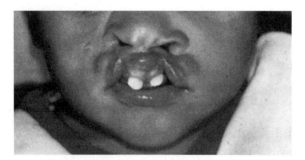

FIGURE 3–7. This child has a severely deficient upper lip and protruding premaxilla. Either of these may interfere with lip closure. This may lead to the use of compensatory adaptations, such as substitution of labiodental stops for bilabial stops, resulting in visual errors but not necessarily acoustic errors.

may be necessary. This is the ONLY situation in which therapy may have to be duplicated.

Visual Distortions

Van Riper (1972) said that speech is defective when it calls attention to itself, interferes with communication, or affects psychological adjustment. This has been interpreted to mean that a speech disorder exists when speech is conspicuous, unintelligible, or unpleasant. The preceding description of compensatory adaptations raises the issue of speech errors that result in accurate sounding but abnormally appearing speech. Some of the adaptations described, such as labiodental inversion of /v, f/ lead to errors which affect how speech *looks*. These are referred to as visual distortions. Nasal and facial grimacing, often produced by speakers with VPI, also affect how speech *looks*, but not how speech *sounds* (Figure 3–8). Some visual distortions correct

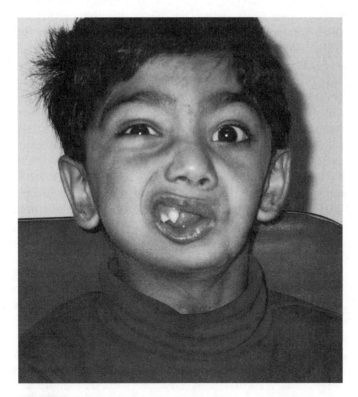

FIGURE 3–8. Facial grimacing is a visual speech distortion associated with VPI. It usually resolves without therapy after VPI is treated.

spontaneously when the underlying cause of the distortion is eliminated. Therefore, the decision to treat visual errors or to wait must take into account the severity of the structural abnormality and whether the correct articulators have been used. If the child has established a habit of using the wrong articulators, as in labiodental inversions, additional treatment may be necessary after physical management. If visual distortions, such as facial or nasal grimacing usually correct themselves after management of VPI, then speech treatment is not needed.

"Cleft Palate Speech" and Compensatory Articulation Errors

"Compensation" is defined in *Stedman's Medical Dictionary* (1976) as "an unconscious mechanism by which the individual tries to make up for fancied or real deficiencies." The errors generally considered "compensatory" in cleft palate speech are glottal stops, nasal snorts, pharyngeal fricatives, pharyngeal stops, and mid-dorsum palatal stops. The first two are usually associated with VPI, pharyngeal stops and fricatives are associated with VPI and palatal fistulae, and the last is more likely to occur in speakers with fistulae. The categorization of all these errors as "compensatory" raises at least two dilemmas. First, although they are all associated with cleft palate, the underlying physiologic deviation is different (fistula vs. VPI). Second, they are not ultimately successful as they severely compromise speech intelligibility. In other situations, when one attempts to "compensate" for a deficiency, attempts are modified if they do not work. For example, a person who loses use of one arm "compensates" by performing tasks with the other arm. A speech example in this category is labiodental inversion by speakers with severe Class III malocclusions, described above. Although compensatory errors work in terms of constricting the air stream, they do not work in terms of producing good speech. Therefore, they should actually be called "maladaptive compensatory errors" (Golding-Kushner, 1995).

A *glottal stop* is a maladaptive compensatory articulation error produced by abrupt adduction and release of the vocal folds. It is usually produced as a substitution for stop consonants, but may be used for other consonant types as well. Glottal stops are phonemic in some languages and occur in some English dialects (as in "ba?l" for bottle). As discussed earlier in this chapter, examination of velopharyngeal motion using nasopharyngoscopy and multiview videofluoroscopy has shown that glottal stop production is accompanied by minimal VP motion in general, and especially with poor motion of the lateral pharyngeal walls (Figures 3–2 and 3–3).

A *nasal snort* is a maladaptive compensatory articulation error produced when the speaker forces air out the nose. It is usually used as a substitution for sibilant and fricative sounds. Nasal snorting is easily distinguished from nasal emission by occluding the nares. If the error is nasal emission, the consonant will be produced correctly. If the error is nasal snorting, the consonant will not create a sound, or will result in a velar sound when the nose is closed, because the intended nasal exit is blocked by the occlusion. Nasal emission is, most often, an obligatory error. Nasal snorting is never obligatory. Riski (personal communication) has suggested the term "anterior nasal fricative" to describe nasal snorting and to differentiate it from a posterior nasal fricative. Nasal snorting is usually accompanied by some degree of nasal grimace, a visual distortion. It was noted earlier that glottal stops are characterized by minimal velopharyngeal motion. This is true even when the velopharyngeal region is fully obstructed by a pharyngeal flap or speech bulb that theoretically provides complete velopharyngeal closure. In contrast, nasal snorting is characterized by absent or outward motion. For example, Figure 3–9 shows the endoscopic view of a speaker wearing a speech bulb that is nearly the full circumference of the pharynx. During the nasal snorting that occurs on attempts at sibilant sounds, the velum and pharyngeal walls move away from the bulb, rather than toward it (Figure 3-9a). The outward movement is necessary to allow the air stream to exit nasally, as intended by the speaker. After a few minutes of therapy using procedures described in this book, the speaker was able to produce an orally emitted /s/, accompanied by normalized movement of the velopharyngeal walls toward the speech bulb (Figure 3-9b).

A *posterior nasal fricative*, also called a velar fricative or velopharyngeal fricative, is a maladaptive compensatory error produced by constriction between the velum and posterior pharyngeal wall. It is usually used as a substitution for sibilant or fricative sounds.

A *pharyngeal fricative* is a maladaptive compensatory articulation error produced by constriction of the vocal tract or constriction between the retracted tongue and pharynx to create frication. It is usually substituted for fricatives, and is associated with both VPI and palatal fistulae (Figure 3–10).

A *mid-dorsal palatal stop* is a stop consonant produced by use of the tongue blade to contact the palate in a central region, anterior to placement for velar stops /k, g/ but posterior to placement for anterior /t, d/ (Trost, 1981). Trost pointed out that, perceptually, the boundary between /t/ and /k/ and between /d/ and /g/ are lost. This type of error may occur in speakers with VPI but, more often, is associated with the presence of a palatal fistula and tongue placement for the stop is posterior to the fistula. Stopping the air with a mid-dorsal stop posterior to

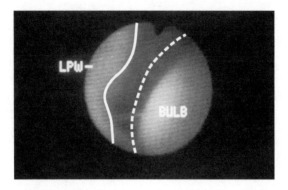

FIGURE 3–9A. Nasopharyngoscopic view of the velopharyngeal region of a large speaker wearing a large speech bulb appliance. At rest, the lateral pharyngeal wall (LPW) is almost in contact with the speech bulb (the position of the LPW at rest is represented by the dashed white line). During nasal snorting, the speaker produces outward motion of the LPW to allow air to be forced out of the nose (the position of the LPW during snorting is represented by the solid white line). From Golding-Kushner, K. J., Cisneros, G., & LeBlanc, E. (1995). Speech bulbs. In R. J. Shprintzen and J. Bardach (Eds.), *Cleft palate speech management: A multidisciplinary approach* (pp. 352–363). St. Louis, MO: Mosby.

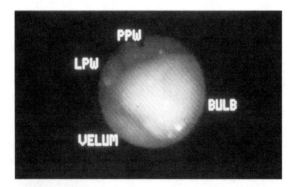

FIGURE 3–9B. The same speaker moves the velum, posterior pharyngeal wall (PPW), and lateral pharyngeal wall (LPW) inward to achieve complete velopharyngeal closure around the bulb during correct oral production of /s/.

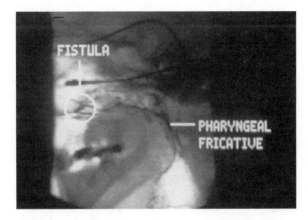

FIGURE 3–10. Image from lateral view videofluo-roscopy showing retraction of the tongue posterior to a palatal fistula resulting in production of a pharyngeal fricative, a maladaptive compensatory articulation error.

the fistula enables the speaker to build up greater intraoral pressure than is possible with tongue placement anterior to the fistula.

A *laryngeal fricative* is a maladaptive compensatory error produced by frication at the level of the larynx. It is usually produced as a substitution for a fricative. It is the fricative equivalent of a glottal stop, in terms of place of articulation.

WHY DO THESE ERRORS OCCUR?

The answer to the question of where speech errors come from is different for each type of error. The etiology of developmental errors may be as much a mystery in individuals with cleft palate as in those with an intact palate. Developmental errors usually represent a maturational delay in control of the small muscles of speech.

The errors considered obligatory are directly related to an underlying anatomic, physiologic, or structural deviation. This can be verified by eliminating the deviation, even temporarily. For example, if a speaker has a palatal fistula and nasal emission, it is often possible to occlude the fistula with pliable dental wax or even with chewing gum and re-test nasal emission. If it is gone, the nasal emission was caused by the fistula.

Adaptations can also be traced directly to anatomic defects, although they are a separate class of errors from those called obligatory.

This is because obligatory errors self-correct when the anatomy is fixed, but adaptations do not. Obligatory errors result in sound distortions, but adaptations represent changes in articulation placement or choice of articulators. Because the speaker has habituated these changes, there is not an automatic reverting to the correct pattern when the anatomic defect is corrected. Thus, obligatory errors do not require speech therapy but adaptations eventually may.

The origin of maladaptive compensatory errors is the least understood. It may be hypothesized that they are an attempt by an infant with an open palate and/or VPI to create the acoustic event of the sound at a place in the vocal tract where this is possible. In the presence of an open cleft palate or VPI, a strong "explosion" of air (hence the term "plosive") cannot be produced. Attempts at plosives are distorted by reduced intraoral pressure and are not acoustically rewarding to the babbling infant. It has been suggested that the infant is aware of their vocal tract limitations by four months of age (Morley, 1972; Lynch, 1986). Also, the weakened plosives may not be recognized by the baby's parents as a plosive, and they will not provide the reinforcement that would normally occur. If, in his vocal play, the baby produces a *glottal* stop, which happens to be a sound produced in all babies' babbling, they may learn to use that for other sound "explosions" as well. Of course, once the acoustic event has been created, there is no need to use the other articulators, leading to the lack of use of the tongue and lips during speech. The glottal sound is reinforced and the habit pattern strengthened. It is, after all, an intelligent and clever strategy the baby learns to get a response. Because glottal stops are not phonemic in English, the sound disappears from most infant sound repertoires very early. However, in some babies with cleft palate, glottal stops may be selectively reinforced and become a learned response to loss of air pressure in the system. Parents may also make a perceptual identification of the glottal stop as an oral sound, and may not reinforce nasalized attempts at other oral sounds because they do not recognize them as oral. The question of why some babies with VPI seem content with weak intraoral pressure and some develop the glottal stops is one that cannot be answered at this time. However, it may be that the maladaptive speech errors result from attempts to avoid or lessen the obligatory errors. The following case illustrates how innocently reinforced glottal stops may become established as replacements for oral consonants.

"How the baby learned glottal stops"

Like most babies, Tiffany engaged in a great deal of vocal play. Because "m" is one of the first sounds to emerge, her babbling started including strings of "mamamamamamama." Very excited, her Mom assigned meaning to her string. "She's saying 'Mama.'" Tiffany tried "dadadada" but it came out as "nanananana" because of an unrepaired cleft palate. Her parents were certain that her next word would be "Dada," and they listened hopefully. One day, she babbled a glottal stop, as do most babies engaging in vocal play, and said "æ-æ-æ-æ-æ-æ." The parents understood this to be the long awaited "dadadada," and became very excited. Baby Tiffany loved the attention and smiles from her two favorite people, and continued to say "æ-æ-æ-æ-æ," which resulted in even more smiles, tickles, and kisses. The Mom and Dad repeated over and over "She said 'Dada,' Hooray for Tiffany!" Unfortunately, the glottal replacement was assigned meaning and received positive attention and reinforcement, and became strongly established as part of Tiffany's repertoire.

THE RELATIONSHIP BETWEEN STRUCTURE AND FUNCTION

In the case of obligatory errors, there is clearly a direct relationship between anatomy and speech error. If there is a leak in the velopharyngeal valve, air comes out the nose. With adaptations, the relationship is usually apparent. The premaxilla is extruded and prevents bilabial closure, the individual produces /b, p/ by creating plosion with the premaxilla and lower lip. However, abnormal structure does not necessarily explain an articulation error nor preclude therapy and it is important to analyze speech errors carefully before attributing them to apparent structural defects. It should not be assumed that errors being made are caused by a structural abnormality that was or is present, even if the error may have had its origin in a structural defect. For example, imagine a child with a severe Class III malocclusion (Figure 3–11) who is unable to say /s/. The SLP must analyze the exact nature of the error. If the child is producing an interdental lisp, it is likely to be an obligatory error. On the other hand, if the error is an anterior or posterior nasal fricative, it is a maladaptive compensatory error, not directly related to the malocclusion. As a rule, maladaptive compensatory errors do not have a direct relationship with anatomic deviations and can be corrected with proper speech therapy independently of medical or dental management. There is, however, an important caveat. Although maladaptive compensatory errors can be eliminated in the presence of anatomic deviations, the therapist, patient, and family must set and understand specific and realistic goals. They must realize that the immediate goal is elimination of the compensatory error, but errors considered obligatory may remain until correction of the structural abnormality. This does not mean that the child will have to re-learn correct production of the sound because, as stated above, obligatory errors tend to correct themselves when the

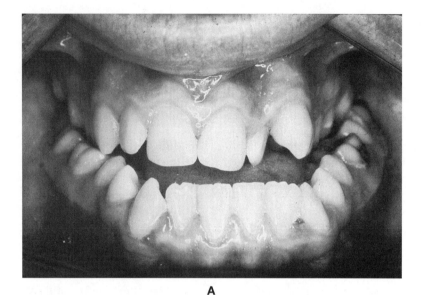

A

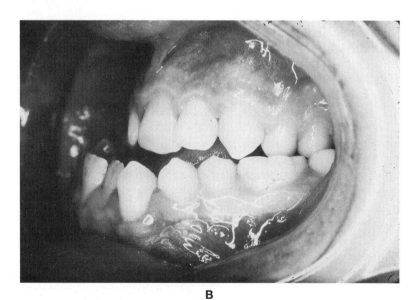

B

FIGURE 3–11A and B. Class III malocclusion seen in (A) front and (B) profile views. Nasal snorting in this speaker is an abnormal compensatory error and should be treated in speech therapy. However, an anterior sibilant distortion is probably obligatory and treatment should be deferred until after correction of the malocclusion.

anatomic abnormality is gone. It does mean that the individual in Figure 3–11 could learn oral production of /s/ and eliminate nasal snorting, but may have an oral sibilant distortion, such as a lisp, until the malocclusion is treated. The justification for treating a compensatory error and "settling" for an obligatory error is the potential for improved VP motion. Speech is also likely to be more intelligible and less conspicuous if the errors are obligatory rather than compensatory.

Unusual Orofacial Anomalies

Individuals with unusual malformations may present with a unique constellation of structural deviations that may contribute to unique speech errors not yet described. Careful analysis must be done to differentiate among errors that are obligatory, adaptive, and maladaptive. If the relationship between the orofacial anomalies and articulation placement/acoustic output is not clear, the assumption should be made that the errors are compensatory, and a short period of diagnostic speech therapy is appropriate until a correct diagnosis can be made.

CLINICAL SPEECH ANALYSIS

We have already said that the compensatory errors produced by individuals with cleft palate are physiologically based. Therefore, they should be analyzed using a physiological model. A traditional approach to sound analysis using a place-manner-voicing paradigm is well suited for this purpose. Phonological analysis examines the sound system on a more abstract level, and does not facilitate treatment planning other than by helping the clinician recognize patterns of sound errors. The astute clinician can recognize certain patterns by glancing at the results of any standard articulation test or speech sample. One does not need a separate procedure to recognize that plosives are replaced by glottal stops, or that final consonants are frequently omitted. Analysis of errors in place of articulation, manner of production, and voicing contrasts provides a physiologically based framework for selection and sequencing of sound and sound-group targets for treatment. This is discussed in greater detail in Chapter 9.

VPI AND HYPERNASALITY

There is not a direct relationship between the severity of velopharyngeal insufficiency and the severity of hypernasality. Many other factors affect the perception of hypernasality such as precision of articulation, degree of mouth opening, nasal obstruction, characteristics of the vocal tract, respiratory and speech effort, and palatal fistulae. Therefore, no assumption about VPI can or should be made based on the perceptual evaluation of hypernasal resonance. Similarly, aerodynamic measures and resonance measures, such as pressure-flow devices and the Nasometer, provide information about a consequence of velopharyngeal activity, and are not specifically diagnostic of VPI.

The only way to diagnose velopharyngeal insufficiency is to look directly at velopharyngeal motion. The most widely accepted techniques for visualization during unimpeded speech are nasopharyngoscopy and multiview videofluoroscopy. During the examination speech production must be taken into account. This is because decisions regarding type and timing of treatment (speech therapy, surgery, prosthetics) are dependent on the presence, absence, nature, and consistency of speech errors, and the consistency of velopharyngeal motion.

WHEN VPI IS NOT REALLY VPI

Special mention should be made of a speech pattern diagnosed as "phone specific VPI," "sound specific VPI, " "functional VPI," "isolated nasal fricative," or "isolated nasal snorting." The terms refer to the situation in which the speaker achieves velopharyngeal closure on almost all speech sounds except for one sound (usually /s/) or class of sounds (usually sibilants). Resonance and nasal emission, when assessed during phrases not containing the error class of sounds, is within normal limits. Individuals with this error pattern are using the velopharyngeal valve incorrectly as an articulator. This is caused by an error in learning but, unlike the maladaptive compensatory errors described above, it is not related to a deficiency in velopharyngeal function. It is essential that this type of nasal airflow be recognized as a sound substitution and not the result of VPI. It is an articulation error that is very easily corrected with speech therapy using the same techniques.

CHAPTER

Getting an Early Start: Infants and Toddlers with Cleft Palate

It should be obvious that when you have a child for a patient, you really have two patients, the child and the parent, who is the primary reinforcer of the child's behavior. Therefore, any intervention that involves babies, toddlers, and children must include the parents and caregivers. Consistency with all adult caregivers is important, and the parent who works most closely with the clinician should convey information to the other adults in the child's world.

The first contact between SLPs and the family of a baby with cleft palate often occurs in the newborn period because of feeding concerns. In most cases, minor adjustments in positioning of the baby and the nipple are successful in establishing a normal feeding routine. In this chapter, we will also consider early intervention, home programs, and the prevention of compensatory errors. Parents should be reminded to follow up with good medical and good ear care, especially because of the high frequency of middle ear disease among children with cleft palate.

FEEDING

Breast Feeding

Babies with isolated cleft lip can breast feed if the breast is placed in a position that allows the infant to create a seal on the breast with the intact part of the lip and alveolus. Most babies with cleft palate have difficulty breast feeding, but can be bottle fed easily and without special equipment or appliances. Some mothers choose to express milk and feed it to the infant by bottle, at least for a short time.

Bottle Feeding an Infant with Cleft Palate

Bottle drinking is usually dependent on the baby's ability to create a lip seal around the nipple and to create an intraoral vacuum allowing movement of the tongue to draw liquid out. This process usually occurs in a simple and rhythmic manner when a baby has an intact lip and palate. When the palate is cleft, the baby's ability to create an oral vacuum is hampered, and this is the main factor that may interfere with feeding. However, successful bottle feeding can usually be accomplished with attention to the position of the infant, the position of the nipple, the opening in the nipple, and keeping air out of the stomach (Table 4–1). The baby should be held in a relatively upright position, either in the crook of the feeder's arm or propped against the feeder's knees, so that baby and feeder are face to face (Figure 4–1). This allows gravity to assist the downward flow of milk when the baby swallows.

The nipple must be placed against tissue, not in the cleft opening (Sidoti & Shprintzen, 1995). That is, if the cleft palate is central, the nipple of the bottle should be placed toward the side of the oral cavity where there is a ledge of intact tissue, rather than toward the middle. In a wide, bilateral cleft palate, nipple placement may have to be between the cheek and alveolus. This placement allows the infant to press the liquid out, rather than draw it, which requires a vacuum-based suction. Placement near intact tissue allows the baby to use a tongue press action to squeeze out milk and keeps the nipple out of the nasal cavity.

TABLE 4–1. *Successful Bottle Feeding of a Baby with Cleft Palate*

1. Hold baby in as upright a position as possible
2. Place nipple in the mouth between two areas of intact tissue
3. Use a softened nipple
4. Use a cross-cut nipple
5. Stop feeding to burp baby at frequent intervals of 5 to 8 minutes
6. Limit feedings to 20 to 30 minutes

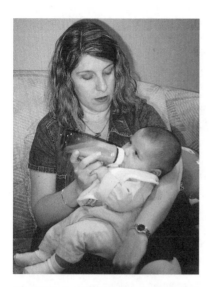

FIGURE 4–1A. Held in the feeder's arm. Note additional elbow support and stability provided by a large pillow.

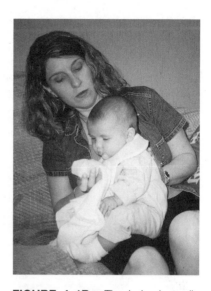

FIGURE 4–1B. The baby is easily moved to a full upright position for burping. Breaks should be taken every 5 to 8 minutes to burp the baby and expel excess air from the stomach.

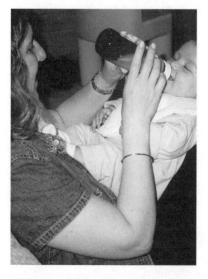

FIGURE 4–1C. The baby's back, neck, and head can be supported on the feeder's raised knees allowing the baby and caregiver to face each other . . . making the baby very happy

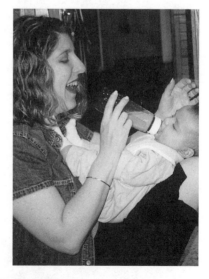

FIGURE 4–1D. . . . . Mommy, too.

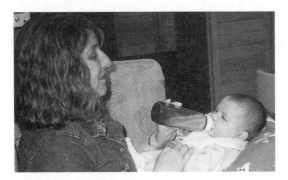

FIGURE 4–1E. Baby can be propped upright against a booster on the feeder's lap, encouraging face-to-face interaction and sound play between drinks. Mom sustains /mmmmm/ . . .

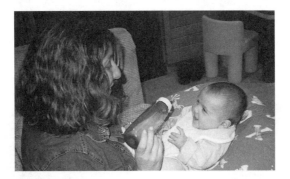

FIGURE 4–1F. . . . which baby finds very pleasurable.

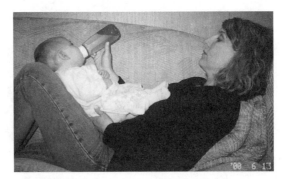

FIGURE 4–1G. Supporting the baby on raised knees while reclining is a favored middle-of-the-night feeding position.

Babies with cleft palate usually do not have dysphagia, or swallowing problems, unless a neurological problem also exists. Therefore, for most babies with cleft palate, swallowing does not pose a problem once the baby has extracted milk from the bottle. Nasal regurgitation may occur but usually diminishes with time if the baby is held in the position described.

Use of a soft preemie nipple or a standard nipple that has been softened by boiling it several times often helps with milk extraction. The amount of pressure needed to draw milk from the nipple may be reduced further by making a crosscut in the nipple using a straight edge blade or scissors (Figure 4–2). The hole should be of a size that allows individual drops to fall when overturned (Figure 4–3 and 4–4).

The final adjustment in the feeding process has to do with burping. If the baby's stomach is allowed to fill with air, it may cause a feeling of fullness before the end of the feeding and may cause discomfort or vomiting. Therefore, feeding should be stopped at frequent intervals of about every 5 to 8 minutes for burping. The feeding should last 20 to 30 minutes at most, in order to insure that the baby is not expending more calories eating than he is ingesting. The interested reader may obtain more information by reading the excellent, detailed discussion about feeding infants with clefts by Sidoti and Shprintzen (1995).

Why should the baby and parent work so hard? Isn't it easier to use a syringe and get the milk to the baby's throat?

The simple adjustments in nipple opening, nipple position, baby position, and burping allow the baby to use the lips, mandible, and tongue in a relatively normal way, without bypassing the oral movements that continue to mature for later feeding skills. The baby may be less likely to become hypersensitive to textures placed in the oral cavity. More importantly, the simple feeding adjustments described allow the parent and baby to engage in the business of feeding in a completely "normal" manner, not made complicated or cumbersome by appliances, special bottles, or tubes. This has the immediate benefit of helping the parents recognize that the cleft palate is something that their baby *has,* not something that their baby *is.* It allows the parent and infant to focus on other crucial things that occur during feeding time. Once the primary goal of nutrition is being met, feeding time is a time of nurturing and bonding. Parents normally sing and talk to their baby during feeding. Parents say that one of the most difficult things about having a very sick baby is not being able to hold them for feeding. One of the saddest sights at baby homes and orphanages in Eastern Europe is a room full of infants being fed by bottles propped up on pillows. They are being fed but not nourished.

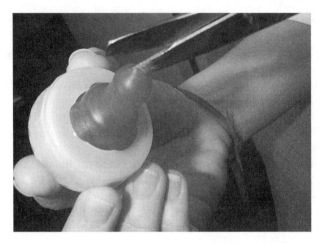

FIGURE 4–2.   A cross-cut can be made in the nipple using a straight edge blade or scissors. This allows the baby to draw fluid out more quickly without pouring it out of the bottle.

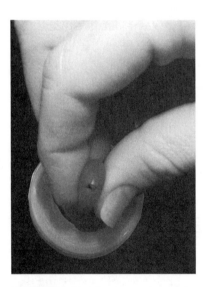

FIGURE 4–3.   Cross-cut in nipple. When the nipple is squeezed, the hole can be seen to have been enlarged slightly.

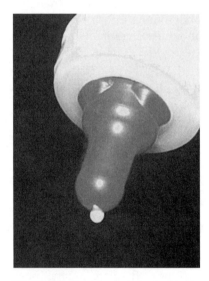

FIGURE 4–4.   The hole in the nipple should be of a size that allows individual drops of fluid to fall when over-turned.

Being held during feeding provides both the caregiver and the baby with the foundation of a close attachment and healthy emotional development (see Figure 4–1). That bonding process is facilitated by keeping the feeding experience as "normal" as possible.

What if the Baby Does Not "Catch On?"

Babies with cleft palate who continue to have feeding difficulties, despite these simple adjustments, are often found to have other disorders that interfere with normal feeding. In other words, it is some other feature of the disorder, not the cleft palate, that is the major cause of the feeding problem. For example, babies with Robin sequence may exhibit feeding problems because of airway obstruction. In velo-cardio-facial syndrome, feeding problems may be caused by generalized and pharyngeal hypotonia, laryngeal anomalies, or vascular anomalies, such as vascular rings that encircle and compress the pharynx. Other babies may have neurological problems in addition to the cleft palate. When the adjustments described above do not resolve the feeding problems, prompt and accurate diagnosis is essential so that the correct medical and/or surgical treatment can be provided. Oral-motor training and feeding therapy should not be assumed necessary until the possible anatomic and physiological deviations requiring medical intervention have been examined and treated.

Feeding and Speech Development

We have seen that feeding and speech are both functions of the vocal tract. If a child has problems with one of these functions, they may have problems with another. However, one must be cautious about interpreting cause-and-effect relationships between feeding and speech. This is because feeding and speech are both secondary to breathing. In other words, the primary role of the vocal tract is to act as an airway. For example, Robin sequence was mentioned in the preceding section. Stickler syndrome is a genetic syndrome associated with Robin sequence. A high percentage of babies with Stickler syndrome and Robin sequence experience airway obstruction. The normal pattern is for babies to breathe and nurse simultaneously, but babies with airway obstruction must do so sequentially. It is the breathing problem that causes a feeding problem. The airway obstruction may be severe enough to necessitate treatment with a glossopexy or even tracheotomy. Once the airway problem has been addressed, children with Stickler syndrome usually bottle feed well and gain weight. Interestingly, the babies with the most severe airway compromise may be the least likely to have evidence of VPI or abnormal compensatory speech errors (Golding-Kushner, 1991). Thus, feeding and airway problems do not necessarily lead to speech problems (D'Antonio & Scherer, 1995).

Feeding and Oral-Motor Skills

SLPs trained in oral-motor therapy may be concerned that encouraging press/munch feeding movements, rather than true sucking, inhibits the normal maturation of oral-motor feeding patterns and subsequent speech development. This is not the case. Most infants fed in the manner described eagerly make the transition to solid foods without difficulty, even before the palate is repaired. They gain weight well and establish normal speech patterns. Furthermore, there is a lack of convincing evidence of a direct link between oral function during early feeding and oral function during speech.

One of the pitfalls of the application of oral-motor therapy for children with clefts is that the focus of oral-motor therapy is on component movements, such as differentiated tongue movement, and the coordination of oral and respiratory activity is ignored. Nonspeech oral movements tend to parallel speech, but not duplicate them. Furthermore, isolating oral movements ignores the frequency and complexity of speech movements. Therefore, oral-motor therapy, per se, is not recommended. Instead, babies who are delayed in the onset of sound-making should receive appropriate sound production "articulation" therapy.

EARLY INTERVENTION

Language Development

Children who have nonsyndromic cleft lip and/or palate fall within the normal distribution of intelligence (Richman & Eliason, 1986). There are many reports in the literature stating that children born with cleft palate have delays in language development (Lynch, 1986; McWilliams et al., 1990; Scherer & D'Antonio, 1995). However, it is our experience that most children with nonsyndromic cleft lip and/or palate are no more likely to have language delays than their peers without cleft palate. This means that the presence of a cleft lip and palate, in and of itself, does not predict a language delay, but children with clefts may experience language delays in the same way, and with the same frequency, as children without clefts. The high prevalence of otitis, frequent hospitalizations, and other factors in these groups may present a risk for language delay, and children born with cleft palate should be considered at risk and receive early language evaluation so that delays are not overlooked. Also, children with cleft lip and/or palate may have syndromes with features that do not manifest until later in development. They may be diagnosed as having *isolated* clefting with language impairment, although they, in fact, have a syndromic cleft. Therefore, children with clefts who also have language delay should be examined very carefully at intervals throughout their development to rule out the existence of other anomalies.

It should be kept in mind that the preceding discussion is based on studies of children in the United States. It has been observed that language delays and compensatory speech disorders may be much more common in regions within the US and in other countries in which families are affected by social, economic, and educational limitations. Ysunza (personal communication) observed that in a large population of patients with cleft palate in Mexico City, language delays are "dramatically common." He suggested that this is probably also the case in many centers in Central and South America.

On the other hand, children with isolated cleft palate seem to be at higher risk for language disorders (Richman & Eliason, 1986; Scherer & D'Antonio, 1997). For example, Scherer et al. (1999) reported longitudinal data comparing 4 groups: normal developing children, children with cleft lip and palate, children with isolated cleft palate, and children with velo-cardio-facial syndrome. The children with cleft lip and palate were not statistically different from the normal developing children. The children with isolated cleft palate showed significant receptive and expressive language impairment. The reason for increased risk of language delays in children with cleft palate without cleft lip is probably that "isolated" cleft palate is more likely to be associated with a multiple anomaly syndrome than cleft lip and palate. Language delays can be predicted with a high degree of certainty in certain syndrome groups, most notably velo-cardio-facial syndrome (Golding-Kushner et al., 1985; Golding-Kushner, 1995; Scherer et al., 1999; Shprintzen, 2000). Therefore, all children with cleft lip and/or palate should be considered at risk for language delay and undergo language evaluations at least yearly, beginning by 8 months of age.

Speech Therapy for Babies

The goal of early intervention programs is to diagnose and treat speech and language problems at the earliest possible time, in the hope of minimizing the effects of early delays and disorders. For children with cleft palate, an important additional purpose of early intervention is to prevent the development of compensatory articulation errors and to treat them if they do occur. SLPs have an important role in educating parents of children with clefts about normal speech and language development, and in teaching parents ways to prevent development of abnormal compensatory speech patterns.

Models of Service Delivery

Babies born with cleft palate in the United States are usually eligible for Early Intervention Programs (EIP) at no cost to the family as mandated by federal law. In most states, EIP services are administered by the Department of Health and Special Services. Babies who are considered at risk for developmental problems may be referred for evaluation by a parent or a pediatrician. Babies and toddlers are usually evaluated across multiple domains, including receptive and expressive language, speech production, fine-motor skills, gross-motor skills, cognitive development, and social-emotional development. States have formulas to determine eligibility for free services. The current formula in New Jersey, for example, qualifies a baby for state-funded early intervention services if he or she exhibits a 33% delay in one domain or a 25% delay in two or more domains. It is important to keep in mind that this formula is calculated to determine eligibility for state-funded services. It is *not* a statement of the presence or absence of a delay or disorder. This means that there will be children who *do* have delays and who *should* receive early intervention services, but do not meet the criteria for *free* services. SLPs can help parents understand that difference. In fact, school-aged children face the same issue (presence of disorder vs. eligibility for services) in many school districts, as will be discussed in Chapter 5. Many insurance companies also have restrictions on payment for services. For example, they may only cover postoperative treatment related to medical rehabilitation but not to educational services. They go on to define "speech" as an educational service that should be provided at school. These limitations should not be interpreted to mean that intervention is not needed.

EIP programs should include ongoing parent training and direct interaction with the baby to provide and to model appropriate intervention techniques. When evaluation shows the child to be developing age-appropriate speech and language skills, early intervention should take the form of quarterly reevaluation and ongoing parent education in normal speech and language development. This enables the parents to detect any deviations from the typical pattern of development so that intervention that is more direct can be arranged if necessary. This follow-up may be accomplished by reassessment by the SLP or, if geographically impossible, the parents may be taught to elicit a good speech and language sample on videotape and send the tape to the SLP for review.

If the child is found to be eligible for funded EIP services, the evaluation team will write an Individualized Family Service Plan (IFSP), which contains the skill areas for which services will be received (e.g., speech, language, feeding, gross motor, cognitive), the designated provider (e.g., SLP, PT, teacher), specific objectives within each domain, and the approved schedule (frequency and duration of sessions). The IFSP will also state the anticipated duration of the program and date of follow-up, usually 6 months. The IFSP serves a purpose similar to the IEP written for children age 3 and older receiving services at school.

Many states urge that EIP services be provided in the child's "most natural environment," which is usually the home or daycare. Therefore, EIP services are not usually provided in an SLP's office.

The primary role of the SLP providing EIP services to babies with clefts is to model methods of stimulation, elicitation, and reinforcement of desired responses for the parents or caregivers who are the child's primary teachers. Parent training also includes providing pertinent information about normal speech and language development. SLPs should provide ear training for parents, so that they can accurately hear the desired speech sounds and detect errors. An advantage to home-based EIP services is that the program can utilize materials already available in the home. This makes it easier for parents to envision ways to make speech stimulation an ongoing, daily activity, rather than a separate and distinct task to be performed at specified times. It is easy for parents to see how speech sound stimulation and language stimulation can be centered on the child's normal routine.

EIP services may be center-based in some communities. When this is the case, parents and babies may have an opportunity for group interaction. This is often beneficial in terms of general language development. However, it has been the authors' personal observation that babies and toddlers who are speech delayed or developing a compensatory speech disorder benefit more from the articulation modeling provided by trained adults than by other language delayed or normally developing babies. Therefore, individual intervention is recommended for babies with clefts, especially those who have speech production issues.

In many places around the world, early intervention services do not exist. Even in the United States where services are mandated, they may not be available for various reasons. When families have limited access to speech and language services for their young children, SLPs may have, at best, limited opportunities to train parents to work on their own as surrogate clinicians. In this situation, active participation of the parents during the speech intervention sessions that can be scheduled with the clinician, and training to allow parents to carry out procedures at home, is even more important. In fact, parent training and participation is critical (Pamplona & Ysunza, 1999b; Pamplona et al., 1996).

Prevention of Speech and Language Disorders

It is easier and more efficient to prevent the development of speech and language problems than to treat them when they occur. Therefore, the focus of early parent training should be on normal speech and language development and on the prevention of delays and disorders. Language and articulation may be addressed simultaneously. The parent should understand that receptive and expressive language skills relate to the symbolic function of communication and that speech refers to the motor aspects of communication—articulation, fluency, and voice. Clinicians should apply their knowledge of normal language development and share information on the expected sequence of development of communication skills with parents. Parents should understand that, even when a particular goal relates to improved speech production, the task occurs within a linguistic context. In other words, even when language and speech are being "treated" separately, they are intertwined and, to some degree, dependent on each other.

Home Programs for Early Intervention

VPI cannot be accurately diagnosed until the child can produce a sufficient speech sample and cooperate for videofluoroscopy and nasopharyngoscopy during speech (Shprintzen & Golding-Kushner, 1989; Shprintzen, 1990). However, articulation errors associated with VPI manifest at the onset of speech, and symptoms of VPI, such as nasal emission and hypernasality, can often be detected by the time the child is attempting several words with non-nasal consonants. Every child with a cleft palate should have an initial speech and language evaluation by 8 months of age, or preferably earlier, when consonant sounds are normally appearing. If consonants do not seem to be emerging, it may suggest that the child is establishing a pattern of glottal stop articulation that should be treated at the earliest opportunity. Intervention at this early stage can frequently be provided effectively through the use of home programs that are administered by the parents and caregivers and supervised by the SLP. This is different from home-based services described above, which are provided by the SLP on a regular basis. In those, the parent's primary role is to participate and work with the therapist, and learn to provide opportunities for practice. In a home program, the clinician is available for consultation, training, and periodic follow-up, but the parent is the primary service provider.

The goal of this very early speech intervention is to reduce the likelihood of the establishment of abnormal compensatory errors as a habit pattern before it occurs (Golding & Kaslon, 1981). This can be accomplished concurrently with early language intervention if the latter is necessary (Scherer, 1999).

Home programs must be individualized to take into account the needs and development of each child and the resources, in terms of time and ability, of the parents to carry out the program. Certain program components should be included in any program. These components are:

1. Evaluation
2. Parent training in
   a. Normal language development and sound production
   b. Recognizing the difference between oral and compensatory articulation
   c. Techniques for stimulating language development
   d. Techniques for eliciting correct, oral consonant production and extinguishing glottal stops
   e. Application of behavior modification techniques
   f. Trouble shooting
3. Follow-up
4. Reevaluation
5. Revision of goals, continued parent training

Evaluation

Receptive and expressive language skills and sound production skills should be assessed by 8 months of age. This age is optimal so that the emergence of glottal stops or other maladaptive compensatory sounds can be treated before strong habit patterns are formed. In babies with early consonant attempts, it may be wise to evaluate sooner. This is because it is easier to prevent the development of glottal consonants than to eliminate them once present. The procedure for evaluating emerging language skills is not different for a child with a cleft than for other children. Many standardized tests which rely on a combination of parent interview and observation of spontaneous and elicited responses from the child are available, including the *Sequenced Inventory of Communicative Development* (Hedrick et al., 1984), the *Infant-Toddler Language Scale* (Rossetti, 1990), and the *Pre-School Language Scale—3* (Zimmerman et al., 1992). *The MacArthur Communicative Development*

Inventory: Toddler (Fenson et al., 1991), which depends only on parent interview, may be useful for language screening when full evaluation is not possible or prior to evaluation to assist the clinician in selection of the most appropriate tests (Scherer & D'Antonio, 1995).

Patterns of language impairment vary among subgroups of children with cleft palate who have multiple anomaly syndromes. In such subgroups, cleft palate is only one of a number of clinical manifestations that may result in a speech or language impairment. For example, in his compendium of approximately 160 syndromes with speech and language impairment, Shprintzen (2000) cites 75 syndromes with cleft palate as a clinical feature, the large majority of which have language impairment as well. The language delays that occur in the syndromes with cleft palate also occur in other populations familiar to speech-language pathologists. Therefore, a language assessment for a baby or toddler with a cleft palate is not different from a language assessment for a child without a cleft palate. On the other hand, the sound production errors exhibited by some individuals with orofacial anomalies are not usually found in other clinical groups. Because of the unique types of errors associated with cleft palate and the interrelationship between compensatory sound production and velopharyngeal function, early speech evaluation in individuals with cleft palate is especially important.

The distinction between language and articulation made throughout this book may seem contrary to the current view that working on language results in improved speech, especially in young children. A recent study even made that point by showing increased phonemic repertoire for a very small group of toddlers with cleft palate who received language intervention (Scherer et al., 1999). The authors suggested that the distinction between language and speech in young children is not clear. However, it is the experience of most clinicians with vast experience working with these children that the distinction is important. Language provides the message transmitted by the speech signal, but it is the mechanics of speech production that are in error when compensatory errors are produced and that need specific and direct treatment.

Parent Training

Home programs for infants and toddlers are effective ways of encouraging oral consonant development and avoidance of abnormal compensatory errors, such as glottal stops. The SLP has an important role in parent training, keeping in mind that parents and caregivers are children's first and most important teachers. The SLP should be skilled in parent training so that the parents can learn to provide appropriate stimulation, modeling, and reinforcement on an ongoing basis. Parents and other caregivers are in a position to provide the type of constant stimulation that cannot be approached by SLPs who spend, even under the best of circumstances, no more than an hour or two per week with the child. In fact, as stated earlier, a number of recent studies have suggested that parent participation in treatment is essential (Pamplona & Ysunza, 1999b; Pamplona et al., 1996).

The first step in training parents to work with their babies and toddlers is to teach them stages of both normal language development and normal sound production. In most families, one parent receives direct training from the clinician. Parent education begins during the initial evaluation and should be kept simple. Parents should be provided with written material for reference to reinforce and supplement information received verbally, such as a chart listing the sequence of achievement of receptive and expressive language and speech milestones. It is natural for parents to compare their child's development to usual ages of mastery, and while parents should know what to expect at different ages, the emphasis should be on the usual *sequence* of mastery. Parent training is ongoing. It is important to convey to the parent that it is his or her responsibility to train the other parent *and* any caregivers that are with the child on a regular basis.

The next area of parent training is in techniques for stimulating continued language development. Parents should be taught how to repeat and expand the child's utterances. Parent-child communication, especially at this early stage of development is often, unfortunately, parent-directed, with an emphasis on requests for naming objects ("What's this?") and locating objects ("Where's the _____?"). This is especially true when the child tends not to elaborate on a topic during a conversation or initiates communication infrequently, patterns exhibited by children with language delays. Parents should be taught to engage in child-centered and child-directed communication. The clinician should demonstrate effective ways of eliciting desired verbal responses by repeating the child's vocalizations and giving the child opportunities to repeat their simple vocalizations, by modeling play behvaior with role playing and other similar strategies. When the parents learn the strategies for interacting in a child-centered, nurturing way, it is likely that they will begin to use these strategies during meals, bath time, shopping, and other events. While the parents may not have set aside a specific time of day to "practice" speech and language, they will have used the facilitation techniques as a natural part of their interactions with the child throughout the day.

When the child will not be seen by the clinician on a regular basis, this training may take place at the time of the initial visit and by using written material. When the child is receiving early intervention services on a regular basis, the parent training can be ongoing and parents can learn by working together with the clinician during scheduled sessions. Additional suggestions that can be given to parents to help them provide full-time language stimulation are listed in Table 4–2.

For children falling into a glottal pattern of sound production, or those not making many sounds, it is helpful to provide the parents with a list of target sounds and words, based on the child's level of language and phonetic development and whether or not the palate has been repaired. Initial target words before palate repair should be vocalic and nasal-loaded with an emphasis on words that do not begin with vowels. This is because vowel-initial words actually begin with a glottal stop. The goal is to teach the child alternate word-initial strategies. Stimulation should be constant throughout the day. The parents should take advantage of every opportunity to interact verbally with the child throughout the day, rather than segmenting separate time to "practice"—this is full time. Very early on, babies can "play" with aspiration, production of sustained "hhhhhhh," and play by overlaying movements on the sustained "hhhhhh" to produce different sounds. Overlaying mouth opening and closing on "hhhh" results in production of /p/. Whispering while laughing is another game, as is saying "shhhhhhh" with the nose closed. Nasal occlusion can be lightened and released on alternate "turns." Parents should focus on pressure consonants and ignore the hypernasality. For babies not using their lips, lip-sound play can be encouraged using vowel plus /w/ sequences, such as "ooowow" and "oowee."

Babies often become very quiet immediately after palate surgery because their mouths are sore. They are ready to resume sound play as soon after palate repair as they feel well, usually within a week or two. At that point, words should be plosive-loaded, with anterior plosives introduced first. Examples of some first words are in Table 4–3.

A crucial area of parent education, and one of the most difficult, is auditory training to recognize the difference between oral and compensatory articulation. The clinician can demonstrate correct and incorrect (glottal) production, use tape recorded samples contrasting correct and incorrect productions, and help the parent identify errors in their own child's babbling or early words. Auditory training for the parent should continue until both the clinician and parent are confident that the parent can hear the difference between the desired target and glottal stops or other abnormal compensatory errors. Training should include the use of auditory cues with and without visual cues. This is important to be certain that they can hear co-produced glottal stops which, like glottal stops, should not be reinforced. It is helpful

TABLE 4–2. *Ideas to Help Parents Stimulate Speech and Language Development in Babies and Toddlers*

Use daily, routine activities. Narrate the baby's day and yours all day long using short phrases. Begin with single words, nouns ("Mommy") or verbs ("eat"). Then combine noun + verb to two-word phrases ("Mommy eat", "David laugh"). Then use adjective + noun phrases ("Big car") and three-word phrases combining nouns + verb + adjectives ("Roll big ball") and other three-word phrases.

Teach social words and phrases such as "please"—emphasize "p."

Develop a core vocabulary of words with pressure consonants for specific daily activities. For example: For dressing: shoes, socks pants, belt, shorts. For dinner: plate, spoon fork. For bathing: soap, etc.

Watch a favorite videotape together and listen for certain words. Sing along with the tape.

Read to the child. Face the child so they can see how you say the sounds.

Read picture books to a 1-year-old using one or two words per page. Increase length of the sentences you "read" as the child's vocabulary increases. Use books that are developmentally appropriate for the child. The same story book can be "read" in a different way for different levels. Be creative in your reading. "Read" the pictures to tell the story using single words then two to three word phrases. Do not think that you must read the written text. The child won't notice until they are much older.

Read books with rhyming words. Leave out a word and let the child fill it in.

At 2–3 years of age start teaching letter recognition to incorporate oral pressure sound production goals with language stimulation. Start with pressure consonants such as "d" for "daddy."

to give the parent a copy of an audiotape to take home so they can remind themselves of the difference when they are at home, and also to help them in his training of other caregivers. When possible, the audio training tape should include their child's sound productions contrasted with the clinician's productions.

Once they can hear the difference between correct and compensatory articulation, parents can be trained in techniques for eliciting correct oral consonant production and extinguishing glottal stops using behavior modification techniques. They should learn to elicit target sounds in words and to provide positive reinforcement when the sound is correctly produced in a word or correctly babbled. Behavior modification technique uses three types of contingency responses—positive

TABLE 4–3. *Sample First Target Words*

Prior to palate repair:	Following palate repair:
Hi	Baby
Hello	Boy
Hey	Barney
Honey (can be name given to a doll)	Pop
Mommy	Pooh
More	Pie
Me	Toy
No	Doll
Whoa!	Cookie
Wow	Go
	Good
	Good girl/ good boy

reinforcement, negative reinforcement, and punishment. Positive reinforcement, which acts as a reward, increases the likelihood that a behavior will be repeated. Positive reinforcement is social in early home programs, and may consist of smiling, tickling, or clapping. The opposite of positive reinforcement is punishment. Punishment is the application of an adverse response to a behavior. It is intended to decrease the likelihood of the behavior being repeated. However, it draws attention to the behavior and the attention itself may, inadvertently, be reinforcing. This is the basis for the advice given by child rearing experts to ignore tantrums. A child having a tantrum wants attention—*any* attention. A child who is having a tantrum and receives attention is likely to continue to have tantrums. On the other hand, tantrums become less and less frequent if they are ignored, and the child learns that having a tantrum is not worth the effort, and stops having them. Therefore, punishment is not recommended for use as part of early home programs. When a behavior is ignored, the likelihood that it will be repeated is diminished. When a child in the early stages of speech development of babbling and reduplicated syllables produces a compensatory speech sound, the production (not the child!) should be ignored. The lack of a response from the parent acts to decrease the likelihood that the undesired sound will be repeated. The parent should be trained to continue engaging in the task with the child, but not respond to the incorrect vocalization. The parent should continue to produce the target sound, exaggerating the aspects of the child's production that need to be corrected. An example of this type of exchange is in Table 4–4.

A special challenge for parents may be learning the difference between speech *intelligibility* and speech *accuracy*. When a child is learn-

TABLE 4–4. *Modeling Production of /p/*

The mother and daughter are sitting on the floor playing with bubbles. Mom is blowing bubbles, and both mom and child try to pop them. Mom reaches for the bubbles and says "Pop!" each time she pops one.

Mom: Pop!

Mom: Pop!

Mom: Pop!

Child: ah

Mom: p^{hhhhhhhhhh}op (Demonstrating initial /p/ lip closure and release with over-aspiration)

Child: ah

Mom: p^{hhhhhhhhhh}op

Child: p^{hh}op!

Mom: (smiling) Yes, p^{hhhhhhhhhh}op You said "p^{hhhhhhhhhh}op"

Mom: (pops another bubble): p^{hhhhhhhhhh}op

ing that his words and sounds can control the behavior of others, it is important to reinforce his communication attempts. This may pose a significant dilemma, especially if the child used glottal stops in his speech but his communicative attempt was successful because of intonation, vowels, syllabification, pointing, and/or gesturing. For example, we know of a toddler whose favorite expression was "uh-oh." This was the only utterance that was intelligible to the parents. They thought it was cute, and repeated it back to him providing constant reinforcement for the utterance. What they did not realize was that both syllables are initiated by glottal stops. Because the child's other utterances, which contained attempts at other consonants, were not reinforced, they dropped from his repertoire, leaving only the glottal stops. A more useful response would have been to modify his exclamation with some other utterance, such as "my, my, my," or "fall down." This might have encouraged him to try other utterances besides "uh-oh."

Finally, parents should be trained in the art of trouble shooting. They should be able to identify and avoid behaviors in themselves that elicit inappropriate or avoidance responses in their child. Parents should learn to recognize the way that their verbal and nonverbal behaviors influence the child's responses.

Follow-up and Reevaluation

Parents should be contacted by telephone every 2 weeks, and the infants should be scheduled for clinical reevaluation every 3 months during the first year. When this is not possible, the parents may be asked to send videotapes of their play sessions with the child on a regular basis. This is useful for monitoring the child's continued speech development and for observing the parent's interactions, so that additional suggestions may be made. It also allows the clinician to see the types of activities that are most effective with a particular child, so that they can be integrated in subsequent visits.

Does Every Child with a Cleft Palate Need Early Intervention?

We cannot predict which children will learn to speak normally and which will develop compensatory errors. Therefore, the parent education program should be provided to all parents of babies with cleft palate because it may enable them to prevent the development of glottal speech. Home programs for elicitation and reinforcement of sounds, such as the one described are *not* necessary for the majority of infants with cleft palate who develop normal speech without intervention. On the other hand, early intervention programs are important for babies and toddlers who have demonstrated evidence of a language delay or who are not producing oral consonants. EIP is also of great importance to children at high risk for language delays and/or compensatory articulation because of a syndromic diagnosis, such as velo-cardio-facial syndrome. Early home-based treatment is helpful for children who *are* developing a glottal pattern of speech, especially when the program begins during babbling and before or at the time of emergence of the first words. In most cases, trained parents working at home are able to elicit normal sound production patterns in their children so that glottal speech is not established and subsequent speech therapy is not needed (Golding & Kaslon, 1981; Hoch et al., 1986).

Use of Parent-administered Home Programs with Older or More Verbal Children

The home program described has been useful with babies who are babbling and attempting some single words. We have seen children at this stage establish good oral consonant production, even though their early babbling and single words contained only glottal stops and vowels. In other words, the home program was effective in preventing compensatory speech from developing and in alleviating a compensatory speech disorder at its emergent phase. Unfortunately, it has not been as successful with children who already had an established phonetic repertoire including glottal stops, even when they were as young as 2 years old or producing two-word combinations. Therefore, most children who are 2 years old or trying to combine words and producing glottal stops need direct articulation therapy, usually provided by the speech clinician.

The parent's critical role in this type of therapy is to carry out short, daily practice assignments. Therefore, the clinician should continue to work with both the child and parent, recognizing that they are a "package deal." At no time should the parents think that their presence is unnecessary. The parents must be present for at least part of each session so that they can carry out the daily practice sessions. They should become therapy assistants, so that the child can receive treatment on a daily basis.

Eliciting Oral Sound Production in Very Young Children

The focus of early sound play should be on production of open sounds, nasal sounds and front sounds. Starting at 2 or 3 months of age, even before they make recognizable speech sounds, babies naturally engage in nonspeech sound-making activities such as lip smacking and making raspberries. These sound-making activities, which use the front of the tongue and the lips, should be encouraged. Lip and tongue play should especially be encouraged when the baby and parent are face to face and during pleasurable activities. Parents are the best judges of their child's happiest times, which is when they will be most receptive and responsive to sound play. These times usually include bath time, diaper and dressing time, and feeding time. The parents should take advantage of these opportunities. Of course, raspberries may not be the best choice of games during feeding!

Nasal Escape of Air and Hypernasality

Sound play should be done with the nares open and closed as early as the baby will tolerate it, even before palate repair. Most babies accept nasal occlusion if it is applied gently, slowly, and using one index finger on each ala rather than with a nose "pinch" (Figure 4–5). Babies are nasal breathers and may become distressed the first time their nose is closed. It is important to occlude the nares for very short intervals and only after the young child has inhaled. The clinician or parent can gently run their index fingers along the cheeks until they reach the sides of the nose. This may be incorporated into a game of identifying body parts. While singing a repetitive verse such as "Here we find an ear," the parent can "finger walk" to one of the child's ears, then tickle it, then sing "Here we find a mouth," while finger walking to the mouth, then "Here we find a nose," while finger walking to the nose, gently pressing in the ala, then singing "pa-pa-pa-pa-pa." The child will eventually try to sing along. If the baby's attempt to repeat "pa-pa-pa-pa-pa" results in glottal stops, the parent should change the "lyric" to "ma-ma-ma-ma-ma." When the baby repeats the nasal chain with the nares occluded, a "p" sequence will result. After many productions, the nasal occlusion can be lightened and the parent can provide a plosive stimulus instead of a nasal. This is an example of eliciting a sound the child can say (nasal /m/) and shaping it into another sound (oral plosive /p/). It is important for everyone playing with the child to focus on the variety of sounds used and to realize that nasalization of the sounds is *obligatory* before palate repair. They should have appropriate expectations for the baby's sound-making skills.

If the child does not make a speech response after several trials, the parent may want to incorporate nonspeech lip and tongue sounds, such as raspberries, lip smacking, and loud "sighs" in order to engage the child in sound-making. The audible responses can be reinforced and shaped into speech sounds during successive trials. Practicing making a loud sigh is essentially the same as training /h/.

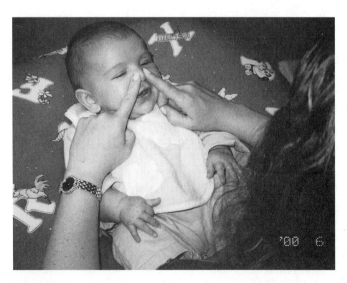

FIGURE 4–5. Nasal occlusion can be achieved for sound play with an infant using the index fingers. This is readily accepted by most infants and does not obstruct the baby's and parent's view of each others mouths.

Some parents may be self-conscious about singing and making up games with their baby. They should be reassured that the baby does not care if they can carry a tune or not. The sillier the songs, the happier the baby, especially if the baby sees that this is equally fun for the parent. Introducing nasal occlusion in the playful way described avoids rapid or seemingly threatening movements, and helps the child learn to tolerate nasal occlusion because the fingers are going to other parts of the face as well. Occluding the nares in this way also prevents obstruction of a view of the babies mouth so that lip and tongue gestures can be seen clearly by the adult, and the adult can be seen clearly by the baby. The clinician and parent should discuss parameters for sound play games with and without occlusion of the nares so that they have a variety of "games." This makes things fun and prevents a dependency on one particular game or setting for a specific speech response.

Parents should be helped to integrate speech and sound play into their ongoing, daily routines and not consider it to be a task that must be practiced at a specific "speech time." They should be taught to "narrate" the child's and their activities using short, developmentally appropriate phrases with emphasis on words containing target sounds, and to engage the child in noise-making lip and tongue play and vocal play at every opportunity.

Baby sound-making should receive one of several responses:

- If the sound is one of the desired sounds, social positive reinforcement should occur and the clinician or parent should repeat the sound made by the child.
- If the sound produced by the child is oral (not glottal) but incorrect, the adult model should repeat the utterance, immediately followed by the presumed target to help shape the child's response. Children make all kinds of sounds, even when a cleft palate is present. Some of these sounds will be oral and those should be reinforced and encouraged, especially when the lips and tongue were used.
- If the sound produced by the child is a glottal stop or other compensatory sound, the utterance should be ignored by the adult model. Avoiding reinforcement may increase the likelihood of extinguishing the specific response.

Special Considerations

The notion of narrating a child's day, talking to a baby, and singing with a baby to provide both language and speech stimulation may be especially difficult for parents who think their baby is not listening, understanding, or responding. There are also cultures in which parents tend not to talk much to babies. In these situations, the families should be helped to understand the importance to the baby of engaging in these types of activities, although they seem awkward to the parents.

Recognizing the First Word Attempts

The shift from babbling to the first words is often a result of the perception of important adults in the baby's world. In most instances, babies do not really say a first word with intention. They babble something word-like, and the utterance is assigned meaning by the parents who are eagerly waiting for these first words. For example, the consonant /m/ is one of the first sounds that babies produce in every language. They repeat it over and over: "mamamamama." At some point, they reduce the number of repetitions and produce reduplicated or double syllables: "mama." The mother, who cannot wait for the baby to "talk," assigns meaning to this syllable combination and, *voilà,* the first word has emerged. It is not a physiological accident that some variation of "mama" has the same meaning in so many languages! In this way, parents guide the attachment of meaning to the child's first words. This process is simple when the focus is on low-pressure sounds and vowels. It is not unusual for a child with a cleft palate to be described by a parent as having a vocabulary consisting of the words, "mama, nana (grandma), wawa, more, nana (banana), nighnigh (night-night), meow, moo, neigh, wow, um hum, ummm, yummy, NuNu (the vacuum cleaner on 'Teletubbies'), hi." These words are readily intelligible to parents.

The glottal stop is another consonant that is babbled by infants in all language cultures. In some languages, glottal stops are phonemic. That is, they are consonants that are used to carry meaning in the same way as /p/ and /b/. In those language cultures, early babbling attempts containing glottal stops are likely to be reinforced as distinct from babbling attempts containing other stop consonants. In English, this is not the case. The child is, instead, perceived as "omitting" consonants.

The production of a variety of consonants and words can be enhanced by recognizing and reinforcing all the baby's oral sound attempts, even when they are nasalized, as is inevitable before palate repair. The example was given earlier of the child who always said "uh-oh," because it was the only non-nasal utterance understood and reinforced by the parents.

Prevention of Glottal Stop Errors

One of the main goals of early home programs for infants with cleft palate is to prevent the establishment of compensatory speech disorders, especially glottal stops. We have said that babbling glottal stops is a natural part of infant vocal development. How, then, can we prevent them from becoming the predominant consonant? Using principals of behavior modification and operant conditioning, the glottal stops should be ignored. It is difficult to conceptualize ignoring an utterance without ignoring a child, but this is what must be done. As we have said, at this very early stage of development a baby is likely to repeat a vocalization if that vocalization is positively reinforced. If the vocalization is ignored, it is likely to drop out of the baby's repertoire in favor of sounds that receive attention. Negative attention (punishment) is still attention and, as we know, children often repeat behavior that receives negative attention because to them, negative attention is better than no attention. When the baby babbles a glottal stop ("vowel-only") sequence such as "ah-ah-ah," the adult should tack on a consonant and repeat the utterance, "ba-ba-ba." If the child attempts to repeat the adult model, which they often do in this game of "I said, you said," but says "ah-ah-ah," the adult should add the nasal consonant and say, "mamama," and should repeat the sequence several times in a sing-song voice, smiling. This type of modeling and shaping provides reinforcement for the babbling itself and provides a model for more appropriate articulation play. The child and parent should continue to play this game for as long as the child remains interested. The parent, after a few "turns" may change their utterance to "ba-ba-ba," which the child is then likely to attempt. If the result is "ah-ah-ah," that is, glottal, the adult should switch back to "mamama" and then gently occlude the baby's nostrils while continuing to say the nasal sequence. The baby's babble attempt will be shifted to the oral "ba" because of the nasal occlusion, and the child will start to hear and feel the production of the oral plosive.

When to Ignore Speech

Skinner's behavior modification theories teach that if a response is not reinforced, an alternate response will be attempted. When a toddler has some oral consonants in their repertoire, certain expectations can be imposed. If a child can say /ba/, but often uses a glottal stop instead, the adult should ignore the glottal productions. For example, an 18-month-old wants his bottle, which he attempts to call "baba" but instead calls "ah-ah." When he says "ah-ah," the parent should feign lack of comprehension and ask "ba-ba?" The child should be encouraged to keep trying. An important consideration in the parent's response is whether or not the /b/ sound is in the child's repertoire, and if it is well established or emerging. If it is not present or is just emerging, the parent should continue to model the correct response and use the nasal /m/ and nasal occlusion "trick" described above to help the child produce the word without a glottal stop, then give the child the bottle. On the other hand, if the child can say /b/ in syllables and words during therapy sessions, the parents should indicate that they cannot understand the request until the child puts the /b/ sound into the utterance. It is important to let the child know that his communication attempt is appreciated, although his glottal speech is being ignored.

When to Start Direct Therapy

The concept of an early intervention program is not meant to be exclusive of direct speech therapy. If a child does not respond to the ongoing stimulation provided by the parents within 6 months, a more direct treatment approach might be indicated. Treatment should shift to the clinician as the main provider, including parents in the sessions, and providing them with short structured tasks to do on nontherapy days. It is essential that the parents understand that, even if the treatment has shifted to a clinician-implemented approach, their presence during all sessions is necessary. We have seen parents go off to do laundry or other household chores while a toddler was engaged with a clinician. Speech therapy should never be considered a "drop-off" activity or a spectator sport. The parents must actively participate in each session. This enables them to receive ongoing training and demonstrates their involvement to the child. It also assures an easier transition for the child to respond to the parent in a therapist role when the clinician is not present.

CHAPTER

5

Beyond Early Intervention: Models of Service Delivery from Preschool Through Adolescence

In an ideal world, children born with cleft palate, or suspected of having velopharyngeal insufficiency, would be identified during their first year of life, receive early intervention services, and develop normal speech. Unfortunately, this is not an ideal world, and the majority of children born with cleft palate who have speech problems receive treatment at a later age.

At the same time, it should not be thought that all speech intervention in older children and teens is needed as a result of failed or neglected earlier treatment. There are situations in which intervention is not needed until the patient is older and has undergone various types of surgical and orthodontic care. In other words, intervention by the SLP may be needed at various cycles throughout the child's growth and development. In addition to discussing different cycles in which SLPs may be involved in the care of a patient with cleft palate or VPI, we will now consider models of service delivery and aspects of treatment such as venue and scheduling.

THE SPEECH THERAPY TEAM

Most individuals with cleft palate or VPI are (or should be) evaluated and monitored periodically by a cleft palate or craniofacial team. This is the means through which multidiscipinary recommendations are coordinated to provide the best possible care. The SLP plays an important role in communicating and coordinating the patient's speech needs with surgeons and orthodontists on the team, who may make treatment recommendations that affect, and are affected by, speech issues.

Because of geography and other considerations, most patients with clefts receive ongoing speech therapy at a location close to home, often at school. This means that most children with "cleft palate speech" have at least two speech specialists involved in their care, the SLP on the cleft palate team and the local SLP. It is important for the clinicians to establish a cooperative relationship and work as a "speech team" so that the patient's needs can be met (Golding-Kushner et al., 1990). The parents may take the initiative to assist the SLPs in establishing communication. If they do not, the clinician should approach them about it, and explain to them that it is in the child's best interest.

Surprisingly, there are parents who resist communication between the local specialist and the team SLP, especially if the local clinician is at the child's school. This is especially true of some parents who have a child with a syndromic diagnosis, such as VCFS. They are concerned about having a child labeled at school because they think it may lower a teacher's expectations. They insist that the child receive speech therapy as an isolated service and believe that anything that occurs outside of school is not pertinent to school personnel. While it is clear that parents with this attitude believe in their hearts that they are protecting their child, they are not. Parents should be helped to understand that teachers are not interested in labeling for the sake of lowering expectations or anticipating failure. Rather, they are interested in finding the best way to educate each child. In the case of a child with VCFS, knowledge of the diagnosis can enhance the teacher's ability to teach the child because there is a growing body of information about what works best with many children with VCFS. In the same way, school SLPs can do their job with the child most effectively if they can communicate with others who are making decisions about treatments that might affect the child's speech.

PRE-SCHOOL CHILDREN WITH CLEFT PALATE

Children in the United States between age 3 and 5 years who have speech problems may be eligible for services through local school districts under the federally funded Individuals with Disabilities Act (IDEA). In some cases, this may be the first encounter they have with a speech pathologist. Speech services provided through the school differ in many ways from services offered by Early Intervention Programs (EIP). The most serious of these differences is exclusion of the parents from the therapy process when school personnel take over the services. This makes it difficult or even impossible for the parents to act as full-time surrogate therapists and tends to make speech something for the parents to "practice" rather than something they can integrate into their daily routine.

Another difference between speech services in preschool programs and EIP is that, in many instances, the emphasis in the school is on "inclusion" and "in-class support." This means that it may be the philosophy and practice of the school to provide speech "improvement" and language stimulation activities for groups of children in the classroom, rather than the more traditional pull-out articulation and language therapy services that are provided individually or in small groups. Unfortunately, this is not an appropriate model for children with "cleft palate speech." This places a burden on the school clinician, who must persuade the rest of the child study team and the district administration that a particular child's needs cannot be met by the district's idea about what is best socially for the child and economically for the taxpayers. One would think that this task should be easy, given that the "I" in IEP stands for *"Individualized."* Unfortunately, in practice, it may put the parents and clinician willing to advocate for the child in an adversarial position with special education administrators.

This task of individualizing should not be underestimated. The current trend toward inclusion is designed to avoid separating the child with special needs from his peers. The reasoning behind this philosophy is that being with children of all abilities teaches the "normal" children tolerance, and they can provide good speech, language, and behavior models for the child with delays. The social benefits for all the children to learn and play together is stressed. While this is nice in principle, the fact remains that if children with compensatory articulation errors are to learn correct speech, they need intensive, individual articulation therapy three to five times per week. Correcting their speech in the most rapid way will be of far greater benefit to them socially than a slow, protracted speech "improvement" program with several children in a corner of the classroom. The child must be able to focus on the therapy tasks, meaning that he or she should be in a room as free from distraction as possible. A classroom with the child's friends and teacher cannot be made free of distractions for this purpose. Speech therapy areas in schools may be small and cluttered with various supplies, but distractions can be minimized to make the setting optimal. For example, shelves of materials and supplies may be covered with a sheet or other makeshift curtain, windows can be covered, and the child can be seated facing the space made most clear.

Children with compensatory errors should be seen on an individual basis at least three times per week. Working with the child in the classroom, if it is *in addition* to the individual schedule, could have the benefit of bringing the teacher into the therapy process, and should be encouraged, even if it is only for a few minutes after a regular session.

In order to be effective, therapy must be intensive and consistent. As we have said, this means that maximum speech production time should occur within each session and sessions should be scheduled a *minimum* of three times per week with daily home practice. It also means that practice must continue during school holidays and summer vacations.

SCHOOL-AGED CHILDREN

SLPs working in schools often have children with cleft palate, velocardio-facial syndrome, and other syndromes of clefting in their caseloads. When these children have complex speech or speech and language disorders, the SLP may be faced with challenges in scheduling, grouping, goal setting, and treatment implementation. Similar issues arise as those for preschool children. Scheduling needs are the same. Children with maladaptive compensatory speech errors require individual therapy three to five times a week for 20 to 30 minutes at each session. Clinicians may have to be creative and consider nontraditional schedules, such as block scheduling (Van Hattum, 1974; Golding-Kushner, 1995). This level of intensity of therapy is usually needed for 6 to 12 months, at which time there has usually been sufficient progress to return to a more traditional biweekly schedule. It must be emphasized that if a child is in biweekly therapy and not doing well, the solution is *not* to implement a program of oral-motor therapy or to teach signing. The solution is to establish a schedule of more frequent articulation therapy with a daily home program.

The school-based SLP, for preschoolers and older children, should play an important role as a member of the child's cleft palate treatment team. The school clinician has knowledge of the child's speech accomplishments in the therapy setting, and has access to information about how the child is using the new speech skills in the classroom. The clinician should ask the parent to keep her appraised of the cleft palate team's recommendations as it pertains to speech, surgery, and orthodontics. She[1] should be made aware of when the child has appointments with the team so that she can share her impressions with the specialists, either by giving a progress report to the parents to bring with them or by calling the team SLP directly. Unfortunately, school clinicians are often not aware that the child has an appointment with the team until a day of school has been missed, at which time it is too late. This situation can be avoided if the clinician and parent maintain regular contact. The clinician will know what other treatments are being considered and scheduled, and the parent will know what the child is learning in therapy and how to practice effectively at home. Parents are often resented when they try to assume the role of coordinator, with the unfortunate result of placing them in an adversarial position with school, speech, and medical specialists. In contrast, parents are the adults who know the child best, and are in the most natural position to maintain contact with each of the specialists caring for the child. By keeping them in the speech therapy "loop," the SLP can empower them to help coordinate the child's care in a positive way.

There are also school districts in which issues of confidentiality and "turf" issues present obstacles that make it difficult for the school clinician to contact an outside team, even with the parent's permission. When working in a public school, this author was once instructed and warned not to contact any doctor directly to discuss surgery or anything else. The reason was that a discussion of that nature had to go through the school nurse, who knew nothing about the subject. This is not mentioned to discourage SLPs, but rather to encourage school-based clinicians to take a more active role as part of the child's "speech team."

THE SLP AND ADOLESCENTS OR ADULTS WITH CLEFT PALATE

SLPs may work with teens and adults who, for various reasons, did not have access to adequate speech services when they were younger. The habit patterns of these more mature speakers are strongly ingrained, as is their self-image as a poor speaker. If they continue to have compensatory errors in spite of earlier treatment, they come to the new setting with a defeatist attitude and an expectation of failure.

---

[1]Although both men and women may be speech pathologists the reality is that most SLPs, especially working in schools are female. The use of the feminine pronoun in the book reflects that fact. It is not meant to exclude or offend anyone, it's simply intended to increase the readability of the text.

For these teens and adults, lack of motivation and poorly developed self-monitoring skills simply add to the challenges affecting their younger counterparts.

Adolescence and early adulthood is a time during which surgical procedures such as maxillary advancement may be done. In some cases, treatment of certain speech errors may have been deferred until these procedures could be accomplished. Some of these young adults may need speech therapy as a result of the changes these procedures bring to their oral architecture. Therefore, they may be receiving speech therapy for the first time.

FUNDING FOR SPEECH THERAPY SERVICES

Speech therapy services may be funded from a variety of sources. As previously discussed, children from birth to 3 years may qualify to receive services through Early Intervention Programs mandated by the federal government and funded through federal, state, and/or local sources. From age three through eighteen years, services may be funded through state departments of education, with services provided in schools. Children attending private schools are eligible for the same speech and other special education services, although they may, in some cases, be provided at a site other than the child's school. Third party payment may be available through insurance companies. Financial assistance may also be available at the state level through the Department of Health through the federal Medical Rehabilitation Act, which has a different name in each state.

Each of the above programs is designed with specific eligibility criteria. This means that there will be some children who have speech and/or language disorders that require treatment but do not meet the eligibility criteria. The criteria for EIP tend to be limited to severity of the disorder and the number of affected "domains" (language, cognitive, social, motor, etc.). The criteria for eligibility for services at school include both severity requirements and documentation of "educational significance" of the disorder. This places much of the responsibility in determination of eligibility on classroom teachers, who are not all supportive of speech pull-out programs. Teachers may be asked to consider academic performance (reduced speech inteligibility affecting teachers' and/or other students' comprehension of the patient's speech, poor reading, spelling, phonics, following directions, etc.) as well as social issues (self-consciousness or history of teasing about speech, reluctance to answer questions or to speak aloud in class) in establishing educational significance. Ironically, children who are doing well academically and are socially well adjusted may have difficulty qualifying, even in the presence of a significant articulation disorder.

SLPs can play an important role in helping parents understand the difference between having a speech disorder and having a *qualifying* speech disorder. This is a concept that may be difficult for parents to accept, especially in our society which encourages feelings of entitlement for free services. Sometimes, parents, teachers, and the SLP can work together to qualify a student. However, there are times that the student will not be eligible.

A similar dilemma may exist for individuals seeking treatment in private practices and other therapy settings. Individual insurance policies vary widely in their coverage of speech and language therapy services. Some policies exclude all therapeutic services, some offer full coverage. Others limit coverage to a limited number of visits for speech disorders resulting from an illness or accident, but exclude "developmental" disorders or those related to a birth defect. There are some policies that only cover a limited number of postoperative visits, or treatment that is determined by their reviewers to be "medically necessary." It is possible to make a case for the medical necessity of articulation therapy to eliminate compensatory errors prior to a pharyngeal flap, because the surgical recommendation and even the need for surgery may be altered as a result of the therapy. However, insurance companies do not consider establishing speech intelligibility to be a medical necessity. They consider it an educational issue, and often insist that services be delivered through the child's school. Of course, if the disorder does not have educational impact as defined by the local Board of Education, a Catch-22 situation exists. The SLP can assist the parents by writing reports and letters that address the specific needs and rationale for treatment. However, the bottom line is that insurance coverage may not be available. The ultimate responsibility for ensuring that a child receives necessary services is the parent's. It is not the responsibility of the government, school, or private insurer. This often means paying for services out of pocket.

CHAPTER

6

Techniques for the Elimination of Abnormal Compensatory Errors

Speech therapy to eliminate abnormal compensatory errors can be simple and quick. It requires the application of principles of behavior management and operant conditioning, knowledge about the mechanics of sound production and, most importantly, an understanding of which component or components in the sound production process are in error. The first step in planning treatment is administration of an articulation test and analysis of speech sound production in words, sentences, and conversational speech. The articulation test used should have stimuli to elicit production of all vowels, diphthongs, consonants, and consonant blends in the initial, medial, and final position of words. A language sample should be elicited to supplement administration of language tests, and can be used for analysis of speech production in conversation. This is an essential component of the speech analysis because articulation competence, nasal emission, and hypernasality may be different in conversation than at the single word or sentence levels.

Results of the articulation test and conversational speech sample should be analyzed in terms of place, manner, and voicing of the sound. Errors should also be categorized as developmental, compensatory, or obligatory in order to facilitate decisions about the timing of therapy and the selection of appropriate targets in therapy. Phonetic distinctions within categories (pharyngeal stop versus laryngeal stop) may be difficult to hear. These distinctions are not too important in planning therapy because the focus of therapy is on how to produce the target sound correctly and not on the error. However, some distinctions may be diagnostically significant. For example, it may be difficult to hear the difference between a velar stop and a mid-dorsal palatal stop, but the latter may signal the presence of a palatal fistula.

The general principles that should be followed are summarized in Table 6–1 and explained below:

1. *Be sure the patient and parent understand the problem.*
   The process of correct speech should be explained to the patient and parent in terms appropriate to the child's level of understanding, and the nature of the error should be defined. Although a complete explanation is beyond the comprehension of children, even the youngest children can understand that the "cough sound" or the "throat sound" is incorrect and "yucky," and that he/she is there to learn to say "good sounds," "windy sounds," and "mouth sounds."

TABLE 6–1. *Principles for Therapy Planning*

General:
  1. Be sure the patient and parent understand the problem

Sound Selection:
  1. Begin with /h/
  2. Proceed from simple to complex
  3. After /h/, train front sounds prior to back sounds
  4. Use sounds requiring one change of feature (such as place of articulation) as facilitators for new sounds

Making Progress:
  1. Move quickly to meaningful syllables and words
  2. Build a corpus of correctly produced words by using target words that contain only correctly produced sounds
  3. Observe criterion levels when increasing complexity

Reinforcement:
  1. Begin with a fixed schedule of reinforcement
  2. Verbal reinforcement should be specific. Give cues and reinforcement for placement and airflow management
  3. Primary reinforcement (edibles) should be avoided
  4. Token reinforcement and reinforcement activities should be quick and built around drills

---

2. *Break the glottal pattern by introducing gentle whispering or use of sustained /h/.*

   It is easy to eliminate glottal stops by using maneuvers that keep the vocal folds apart, such as gentle whispering, over-aspiration, or the use of a sustained /h/ (Table 6–2). This glottal fricative can only be produced with an open glottis and cannot be produced with a glottal stop. All other oral consonants may be shaped from this sound because they are produced (overlaid) on the outgoing airstream initiated by /h/. To use /h/ as a facilitator, easy oral airflow for /h/ should be sustained and the appropriate oral movements may then be overlaid to produce other sounds. Therefore, /h/ is introduced first to break the glottal pattern, teach easy oral airflow with an open glottis, and to make it available for use as a facilitator for other sounds. The sound /h/ should be targeted first regardless of the individual's age. Then the developmental sequence of articulatory mastery should be considered in the selection and sequencing of sounds. Target phonemes should be maturationally appropriate for the child. In general, treatment begins with /h/ and then proceeds from front sounds to back sounds. Within these parameters, the choice of specific phonemes should be based on results of stimulability testing and begin with sounds most easily produced by the individual.

3. *Move quickly from nonsense syllables to meaningful open (CV) syllables and monosyllabic CVC words.*

   Build a corpus of words in which all sounds are correctly produced. As production of new phonemes is learned, "old" sounds are continuously practiced by their appearance in words of increased phonetic complexity. The advantage of this is that untrained listeners (which includes patients and their parents) often have difficulty focusing on a specific target sound within a word. This may cause confusion in the mind of the patient and parent who can hear that a word is not correct even though a particular target sound within that word is correct. The child and parent may have difficulty distinguishing between the correctness of the sound and the correctness of the word. In order for operant

---

TABLE 6–2. *Procedures to Eliminate Glottal Stops*

---

1. Whisper plosive sounds with over-aspiration, introduce voicing at the end of the syllable with a gradual VOT (voice onset time) shift.
2. Sustain /h/ with labial or lingual gestures overlaid.
3. Produce nasal cognate with nares occluded.

---

conditioning to be effective, the stimulus and response must be unambiguous. An exception to this rule is that some words containing nonpressure sounds, such as /r, l/ in the final position, are linguistically important in a young child's world, and compensatory errors on these sounds in the final position of words are rare. Some examples are the words "more, ball, doll."

4. *Elicit multiple repetitions on each presentation to maximize the number of correct productions elicited per session.*

   Hoch et al. (1986) advocated eliciting a minimum of 100 correct productions per session. This is easily accomplished using modified drills. Repetitions should never occur as isolated responses. Rather, they should be produced in rapid succession, with a minimum of five repetitions per response cycle. In order to achieve the desired 100 responses, 20 different stimuli would be needed. The procedure for sound elicitation with toddlers (2- and 3-year olds) is usually play oriented, and it may be difficult to elicit that many responses. Therefore, a minimum goal of 50 correct responses per 30 minutes is recommended. Specific procedures are discussed in detail in Chapter 8.

5. *Obligatory errors cannot be eliminated therapeutically.*

   Speech therapy is inappropriate and contraindicated for obligatory errors caused by VPI, such as nasal emission and turbulence. As discussed in the previous chapter, other structural abnormalities may also lead to obligatory errors. For example, bilabial closure may be impossible with a severely protruding premaxilla. In these cases, the errors should be analyzed to determine if they represent the best possible accommodation to the anatomy. If they do not, and if physical management will not occur in a short time (6 months) *and speech intelligibility is significantly compromised,* consider teaching compensatory adaptations to enhance intelligibility.

6. *Be direct and specific.*

   Tell the patient exactly where to place and what to do with the lips and tongue, and how to direct the outgoing air stream (Golding-Kushner, 1989; Golding-Kushner, 1995). Directions such as "make the wind come out your mouth" are useful, especially for fricatives and sibilants.

TECHNIQUES FOR THE ELICITATION OF SPECIFIC SOUNDS

The most useful approach uses traditional articulation therapy techniques emphasizing correct place and manner of articulation, with special emphasis on making speech "windy." However, the compensatory errors of this population may require some "special" techniques. Many of the procedures used by the author were based on the pioneering work of Morley (1970) and Van Riper (1972) and are modifications of procedures described previously (Hoch et al., 1986; Golding-Kushner, 1989; Golding-Kushner, 1995). Sound selection requires knowledge of specific features of each sound and the age of acquisition of phonemes (Tables 6–3 and 6–4).

Beginning Therapy: /h/

Treatment of compensatory speech disorders should always begin with /h/. To teach /h/, the child should be instructed to open the mouth wide and sigh, or breathe out. Tactile cues and feedback may be provided by producing the sound onto an open palm. With a young child, the clinician may encourage increased oral air emission by telling the child to "make so much wind that you blow me over." Toddlers are greatly amused by their "power" to knock over a grownup by making a big, windy sigh. When the clinician or parent is satisfied with the easy-onset oral air emission on /h/, they can "fall" over and say "You made so much wind you blew me over!" Another activity to elicit /h/ which young children find fun is to "clean" a pair of play sunglasses with their breath. They use the outgoing oral air in the same way as an adult may try to clean their glasses, although most adults are not conscious of the fact they are actually cleaning their glasses with an /h/. The /h/ should, at first, be produced in isolation so that a whispered, oral air stream is sustained for the duration of the exhalation.

The next step is to produce open syllables with the structure /h/ + vowel (V). This builds the initial corpus of correctly produced words. Because vowels are voiced, it also introduces coordination of respiratory and laryngeal activity by teaching voiceless to voiced transitions. Meaningful syllables can include: hay, he, high, hi, ho, who, huh. If the child is too young to be asking "who?" questions, they may be excited about playing with stuffed animals and making animal sounds. An owl can be used to elicit production of "who." When the simple /h/ + V syllables can be produced, combinations can be introduced to increase the repertoire such, as hah-hah (mock laughing), and hee-haw (elicited using a picture or stuffed donkey). The /h/ should be prolonged prior to initiation of the vowel. If a glottal stop is co-produced or inserted, the entire word should be whispered until it is produced correctly 10 consecutive times. Then another attempt can be made to introduce voicing on the vowels after sustained /h/. For a patient with a severe articulation disorder, the initial word list will be limited and may contain only /h/ + vowel/nasal words (hay, he, hi, high, ho, who, ham, hem, him, her, hum, honey, etc.). Target words available for drill become more diverse as therapy progresses.

TABLE 6–3. *Classification of Consonant Sounds Produced in American English*

IPA Symbol	Sound	Age of Acquisition*	Place of Articulation	Manner	Voicing
Labial					
m	m	2	bilabial	nasal, continuant	voiced
b	b	2	bilabial	stop plosive	voiced
p	p	2	bilabial	stop plosive	voiceless
w	w	2½	bilabial rounding w/out contact	continuant	voiced
f	f	3	labio-dental	fricative	voiceless
v	v	5	labio-dental	fricative	voiced
Lingual: Anterior					
θ	th	6½	lingual (tip)-interdental	fricative	voiceless
ð	th	6½	lingual (tip)-interdental	fricative	voiced
n	n	2	lingual (tip)-alveolar	nasal, continuant	voiced
d	d	3	lingual (tip)-alveolar	stop plosive	voiced
t	t	3	lingual (tip)-alveolar	stop plosive	voiceless
l	l	5	lingual (tip)-alveolar	lateral, continuant	voiced
z	z	6	lingual (tip)-alveolar	sibilant, continuant	voiced
s	s	6	lingual (tip)-alveolar	sibilant, continuant	voiceless

Lingual: Mid					
ʃ	sh	5	lingual (blade/tip)-post-alveolar	fricative, continuant	voiceless
ʒ	zh	5	lingual (blade/tip)-post-alveolar	fricative, continuant	voiced
j	y	4	lingual (blade/tip)-post-alveolar (w/out contact)	continuant	voiced
tʃ	ch	5	lingual (blade/tip) t+sh	affricate (stop+fricative)	voiceless
dʒ	j	5	lingual (blade/tip) d+zh	affricate	voiced
Lingual: Posterior					
ŋ	ng	4	lingual (dorsum)-velar	nasal, continuant	voiced
k	k	3	lingual (dorsum)-velar	stop plosive	voiceless
g	g	3	lingual (dorsum)-velar	stop plosive	voiced
r	r	6	lingual—retroflex w/out contact	continuant	voiced
Pharyngeal					
h	h	2	glottal w/out contact	aspirate, continuant	voiceless
ʔ	glottal stop	glottal	stop	voiceless	

*Age of acquisition listed is the age by which 90% of speakers are able to produce a given sound in the initial word position (except /ŋ/ which occurs only in the medial and final word positions) (Fudala, 2000).

Stops consist of three parts: closure, opening, and aspiration.

The voiced-voiceless contrast in stops in the initial and final word position is produced by variation of the voice-onset time for the following vowel. In the final position, there is less aspiration released following voiced stops.

Vowels

Vowels requiring lip rounding and protrusion are /o, u, ɔ/. Vowels requiring an open mouth are /ɑ/ and /ʌ/. The vowel /i/ (tea) requires lip retraction, /e/ (day) is produced with slight mouth opening and lip retraction. The diphthong /aɪ/(hi) combines the mouth opening for /ɑ/ with lip retraction for /i/. It should, therefore, be taught after /i/. The diphthong /ɔɪ/(boy) should be introduced after /ɔ/ and /i/ (see Table 6–4). Vowels, if distorted, should be trained using C-V (/h/ + vowel or /m/ + vowel) syllables. Vowels should not be trained in the initial position of words because this requires a glottal stop onset. Auditory cueing combined with visual modeling and verbal instruction about lip position is usually sufficient for elicitation of vowels. Therefore, vowels produced with tongue retraction (back vowels) are introduced even though back consonants are deferred until later in therapy. Front and back vowels can be combined with /h/ and bilabial sounds. However, when tongue sounds are introduced, front vowels provide a good phonetic context for tongue-tip sounds and should be used prior to combining back vowels with tongue-tip sounds. Similarly, back consonants /k,g,ŋ/ should be elicited using back vowels and then combined with front vowels.

Front Sounds, Low Pressure

Bilabial Semi-vowel

Another early developing sound is /w/. Like the vowels, this sound is produced correctly most of the time. However, if an individual does not produce it correctly, it should be the consonant introduced after /h/. This is because it has bilabial placement (not closure), is anterior,

TABLE 6–4. *Classification of Some Vowel Sounds Produced in American English*

IPA Symbol	Example	Lips	Tongue Height	Location of Tongue Constriction
u	who	rounded, protruded	high	back
o	toe	rounded, protruded	high	back
ɔ	ball	rounded, protruded	mid	back
ɑ	hot	open	low	back
i	tea	spread	high	front
e	say	spread	high	front
ɛ	egg	open	mid	mid

visible, and does not require velopharyngeal closure. It is, therefore, a sound that most children learn quickly, providing ample opportunity for positive reinforcement and establishing an "I can do it" attitude toward speech therapy. The easiest way to teach /w/ is by asking the child to sustain "oooooooooooo" (as in 'moo') and sliding into "ahhh" (as in 'hot'). The transition from "lip pointing" for the "oo" to mouth opening for "ah" results in production of /w/. If the child omits lip rounding and protrusion for vowels and/or /w/, this is an excellent activity to improve lip use for the sounds. Lip movement is elicited during production of the speech sounds for which the lip protrusion/ rounding is used. This is more effective and efficient than performing lip "exercises" to "improve the range of motion of the lips." Skills trained using oral-motor exercises do not automatically transfer to use of the same movements during speech sound production and are an unnecessary step in the speech therapy process for this population. Most children with repaired cleft lip produce sufficient lip rounding for speech purposes. However, even for a child with a severely scarred and tight lip and protruding premaxilla, it is more efficient and effective to train the vowel and consonant sounds using the lip movement than to do isolated physical therapy type exercises for the lips.

Bilabial Nasal

If the child does not produce nasal consonants correctly, the next sound introduced should be /m/. This follows the principle of working at the front of the mouth first. The reasons for this are to keep the sounds far from the source of the glottal or pharyngeal substitutions and to keep the sounds visible. Instructions for production of /m/ are "close your mouth and hum." It is physiologically impossible to produce a glottal stop when doing this. Also, this sound is opposite /h/ on almost every physiological parameter. Therefore, its introduction after /h/ should not cause any confusion. It is closed, voiced, and nasal whereas /h/ is open, voiceless, and oral. Initial meaningful syllables and words with /m/ + vowel construction are "may, me, my, mow, moo, meow, more." Once the child is able to correctly produce /m/ in the initial word position, it can be moved to the final position in monosyllabic words using /h/ or /m/ in the initial position: "home, him, ham, hum, hem, mom." Medial position /m/ can be introduced in the words such as "hammer, mommy." This illustrates the way in which the corpus of correctly produced words builds on sounds introduced and target sounds are treated in overlapping sequence. If /m/ is correctly produced, the words listed may be included in the child's list of correct words and /m/ does not have to be singled out as a therapy target.

Front Sounds, High Pressure: Bilabial Plosives

The next sound introduced should be /p/. Many young children find it easier to produce voiceless pressure sounds than voiced pressure sounds. This may be because the longer duration of glottal opening for a voiceless sound makes the contrast between the target and a glottal stop greater for a voiceless stop. Also, production of voiced sounds is associated with higher vocal tract pressure than voiceless sounds, meaning that VPC is even more critical for voiced sounds than for their voiceless cognates. During production of a voiceless stop, there is increased focus on aspiration and oral air emission. Production is, therefore, physiologically distant from the glottal stop. Thus, /p/ should be introduced before /b/. This may be done using /h/ as a facilitator. The procedure for using /h/ to elicit /p/ is based on earlier descriptions by Hoch et al. (1986) and Golding-Kushner (1995). To produce /p/, sustain /h/ then close and open the lips. If the laryngeal activity (i.e., open airflow) for the "h" has been continued and not interrupted at the larynx, an oral and aspirated /p/ without glottal stop will result. It is essential to listen carefully to be sure that a glottal stop has not been inserted at the /p⁻/ release, or co-produced. When first introduced, the /p⁻/ release should be over-aspirated. Easy over-aspiration of the sustained /h/ usually breaks the glottal pattern because it requires an open glottis which is in physiologic conflict with the glottal stop. The individual should be told to "make a big 'h'." Using this technique the word "pay" should be produced as /p/ + "hhhay." The easy over-aspiration may be phased out as accuracy increases. The sequence of trials using successive approximations to establish production of the word "pay" might be as follows. Each line is repeated until there are *at least five consecutive correct productions*. This means that if there is an error on the fourth or fifth trial, the count from one begins again. In the example, repeated letters represent elongation of a sound, and the underlined segments are voiced.

p^{HHHHHH}aaaaay   (fully whispered)

p^{HHHHHH}aaa<u>aaay</u>   (voicing is introduced after the vowel onset)

p^{HHHHHH}<u>aaaaaay</u>   (voicing is introduced at the vowel onset)

p^{HHH}<u>aaaaaay</u>   (duration of aspiration is decreased)

p^H<u>ay</u>   (normal production)

The next logical sound to introduce is /b/. If a sound facilitator is needed, either /m/ or /p/ may be used. /b/ differs from /m/ on two features: manner (stop versus continuant) and nasality. It differs from

/p/ only on the feature of voicing. To use nasal /m/ as a facilitator for /b/, ask the child to say a word containing /m/ such as 'ma' and occlude the nares, which will force the exhaled air out of the mouth. Tell the child to continue producing /mɑ/ even after you close their nose. Do not occlude the nose on the first two repetitions, then occlude it. They will produce /b/. Smile and tell them "Keep going." The sound, now a /b/, should be produced ten times in rapid succession without releasing the nose so they have a clear auditory model of their own /bɑ/ production. Then tell them they actually produced /bɑ/ Have them do it again while you hold the nose. If the child reverts to a glottal stop, tell them to practice "ma" again, and hold the nose. As production transforms to "ba" tell them "Now you are saying ba, keep saying it." Calling the sound /mɑ/ instead of /bɑ/ when therapy is beginning is often helpful because if you ask for "ba," the child will usually produce a glottal stop syllable, [ʔa], in which case holding the nose will not help. After ten additional correct /m/-turned-/b/ productions, release the nose. Tell the child they said "ba" 10 times. Tell them to do it again while you hold the nose. Tell them to pretend they are still saying "ma" but to turn it into "ba." Hold the nose and have them do ten repetitions. If there are errors, go back one step again until this step is successfully completed five times (ten correct repetitions five times). That means the child will have said "ba" 50 times. This should take about 2or 3 minutes. The next step is to have them say "ba" with the nose open. Tell the child you will start out the same way, holding the nose, but that you will let go and they should continue making the same sound. Begin the same way, but after the third "ba" release the nares for one "ba", then close them again for the next. Smile and say "Good! You kept doing 'ba'! You made the same sound." If they inserted a glottal stop, drop back one level, then try again until they succeed. On the next sequence, begin with the nares occluded and then release the nose after the second trial. Keep the nares open until there are 10 correct productions of "ba" with the nose opened. It is also sometimes helpful to tell the child to say the sound while "holding" their breath. Of course, this cannot be done because speech occurs on an outgoing breath stream. However, the attempt to hold the breath seems to facilitate production. If the child has an unoperated and unobturated cleft, or VPI, there *will* be nasal emission and reduced intraoral pressure during production of this sound. This is obligatory and expected, and should be ignored. There should, however, be a sufficient contrast with /m/ to be perceived as /b/ by the clinician, child, and parents.

If the child has difficulty establishing /b/ in the initial position of the syllable, it can be introduced in the medial or final position using /m/ as a facilitator and the same technique described. Instead of /mɑ/ the stimulus might be /ɑm/. This procedure may be used to elicit /p/

or /b/. For example, if the child can say "hammer" ask them to repeat it several times. Then, the clinician can close the child's nose as the /m/ is being produced so that it is released orally, resulting in a /b/ or /p/ and shifting the word to "hamper." The next step is to repeat the /p/ syllable that results, as in "hamper – per." The child should be told to "make the sound very windy." This facilitates a rapid shift to production in the initial word position.

To use /p/ as a facilitator for /b/, consider that the difference between a voiceless and voiced plosive is the voice-onset time (VOT) of the adjacent vowel, not the mechanics of the consonant gesture. The child can be asked to produce a "loud /p/." Use of /p/ to elicit production of /b/ would add the following steps to the sequence described above for the use of /h/ to facilitate /p/:

$p^H\underline{ay}$ (normal production)

<u>baay</u>   (aspiration phased out, voice onset introduced earlier,
                                        results in production of /b/)

When /p/ and /b/ are added to the list of sounds produced correctly at the syllable and word level, the corpus of meaningful words that are produced correctly may be expanded to include words, such as pay, pea, pie, Po, Pooh, paw, pa, pear, pail, bay, bee, bye, bye-bye, bow, bow-wow, boo, map, mop, baby, Baby Bop, bear, palm, happy.

Production of oral plosives is easier in the medial or final word position for some individuals. This should be considered in sequencing target sounds and contexts. When medial position seems easiest, /h/ may be used effectively as a facilitator while lip or tongue movements are overlaid on the sustained outgoing air stream. For example, to produce /p/, sustain "h" while closing, then opening the lips. The instructions to a young child are, "keep the wind coming out." This initially results in a whispered "hapah." Voicing is introduced at the end of the sequence until the segment after the lip closure is voiced. Voicing is gradually moved to the first appearing vowel, so that the /h/ and /p/ are voiceless but both vowels are voiced. The following sequence was described by Golding-Kushner (1995). Each step is repeated until correctly produced five consecutive times, as follows. Repeated letters represent elongation of a sound, underlined segments are voiced.

^{HHHHHH}AAAAAA	(fully whispered)
^{HHHHHH}AAA^{PHHHHHH}AAAAA	(fully whispered, bilabial closure overlaid)
^{HHHHHH}AA^{PHHHHHH}AA<u>AAAA</u>	(voicing is introduced after the vowel onset)
^{HHHHHH}AA^{PHHHHHH}<u>AAAAAA</u>	(voicing is introduced at the vowel onset)
^{HHHHHH}AA^{PHHH}<u>AAAAAA</u>	(duration of aspiration at p⁻ release decreased)
^{HHHHHH}AAP^{h}<u>A</u>	(normal duration of p⁻ release for medial position)
^{HH}AP^{h}<u>A</u>	(decreased duration of "carrier aspiration")
P^{h}<u>A</u>	(normal production in initial position)

Tongue-tip Sounds: Low Pressure

Vocalic

The next group of sounds to introduce are tongue-tip /j/ ("y"), followed by nasal /n/ and plosives /t/ and /d/. Most children are able to
produce /j/, but it should be introduced if an individual cannot. Providing a visual model ("watch me") and imitation of an adult acoustic
model are usually sufficient to elicit correct production, which requires
a slight "flip" of the tongue tip, but does not require contact with any
other structure. Children like playing with sound and repeating "yea,
yea, yea." They can provide the chorus for a playful parent or clinician
who sings "I love you—yea, yea, yea" to the tune of the Beatle's "She
Loves You."

Lingua-alveolar Nasal

The nasal /n/ should be the first tongue tip-alveolar sound introduced,
if absent, because it is easiest and the most useful facilitator for establishing the oral plosives with the same place of articulation. The verbal
instructions for /n/ are "open your mouth and put your tongue inside
your teeth." Tongue placement is actually on the alveolar ridge. However, referring to the teeth is a more understandable landmark for
young children. Examples of good early words to introduce with /n/,
adding to /h, p, b, m/ are: no, knee, neigh, new, nah, nine, mine,

money, honey, pin, pan, pen, penny, pain, pine, bun, bin, bunny. Spatial prepositions "in" and "on" are frequently used words with /n/. However, caution should be exercised in presenting vowel-initial words when working on breaking a glottal pattern of speech.

Tongue-tip Sounds, High Pressure: Lingua-alveolar Plosives

To introduce plosives /t/ and /d/, the procedures described for /p/ and /b/ may be applied and modified. Most children respond best to introduction of voiceless /t/ before voiced /d/. To use /h/ as a facilitator, the child should sustain the outgoing air while tapping the alveolar ridge (back of the teeth) with the tongue. This results in whispered "hatahtah." After five consecutive correct productions, voice should be added to the final vowel, and gradually added to the vowels proceeding the /t/ sounds. It often helps to occlude the nares while the child is producing the sequences, and releasing the nares after five consecutive correct productions. Instructions to make the /t/ "harder," "stronger," or "louder" may be used to shape the /t/ into /d/. It also helps to tell the child "Don't turn off your voice, keep buzzing." To use /n/ as a facilitator, nonsense syllables or words pairing the nasal and plosive "-nt" or "-nd" may be introduced. Sample words using phonemes learned prior to this phases are paint, pant, mind, wind, windy, window, behind, around, moment, island, hand, band, pond, handy, Mandy, Monday, Indian, Mindy, panty, hunt. The clinician should tightly occlude the child's nares after initiation of the /n/. Because the child has been instructed to not move the tongue, the plosive sound will be produced. After five consecutive correct productions, the child should be able to produce the nasal–plosive sequence with the nares open. The clinician, acting in a cheerleader-type role, should provide ongoing verbal cues and reinforcement such as "Ok, now make it blowy—that's it, keep your tongue there. Do it again. I heard nnnnnnnt . . . ." If an error occurs, the previous level should be repeated until there are another five consecutive correct productions. The clinician should use the fingers on one hand to count so the child can see the number completed and knows how many are left for the sequence. He or she can quickly see that all productions come in fives. After the child has produced five consecutive correct responses with the nose opened, the word should be produced with the nares occluded for the entire word, resulting in omission of the /n/ and good production of /d/, then with the nose opened so that the child has produced the /d/ without the facilitator /n/. A sample sequence is:

hand (nose closed after /n/ onset 5×)

hand (nose opened 5×)

hand (nose closed for entire word 5×)

had (nose opened 5×)

If cues to "make it windy" are used, a /t/ can be elicited instead of the /d/, resulting in production of the word "hat." At this stage, the child can say "not yet." This can be rehearsed many times a day. It provides variety to their usual "no!"

Back (velar) Consonants

Velar Nasal

The final group of plosives are the velars /k, g/, which are the most challenging because of their posterior placement and physical proximity in the vocal tract to the glottal stop. The most useful facilitator for these sounds is the nasal /ŋ/, which is only produced in the medial and final word positions. Therefore, /ŋ/ should be trained before /k, g/ even though it is a later developing sound. To elicit production of /ŋ/, the dorsum of the tongue must be brought in contact with the velum, *not* the posterior pharyngeal wall. This is critical in order to avoid teaching pharyngeal stops. The phonetic context most likely to facilitate elicitation of velar /ŋ/ is the vowel /i/ because it is produced with the highest tongue position of all the vowels.[1] The consonant should be embedded in the medial position of a VCV sequence: /iŋi/."

If phonetic facilitation is not successful, the child can pretend to drink and make a gulping sound. It is often helpful to pretend to drink with the head flexed, which brings the back of the tongue closer to the velum than a neutral or extended head position. Another strategy is to have the child produce sustained /n/ while the clinician holds the tongue-tip down with a tongue depressor. When this is done, most children respond by bunching the dorsum of the tongue and elevating it toward the palate, yielding a good /ŋ/. The tongue depressor can be phased out as the child learns the correct lingua-velar placement. Words with /ŋ/ to be added to the child's practice list include: hanger, hungry,

---

[1]The high vowel /i/ is referred to as a *front* vowel. The tongue blade is bunched and it's highest point is in closest proximity to the middle of the palate. The vowel /u/ is a high *back* vowel, with its highest point closest to the velum. However, when used to elicit velar consonants, the /u/ context may result in production of a pharyngeal stop instead of a velar stop. If this occurs, the /u/ context should not be used.

hang, hunger, wrong, wing, young. In addition, -ing may be added to verbs in the child's repertoire (/h, m, p, b/), such as "hopping, mopping, popping." The first words in this group should exclude tongue-tip sounds /t, d, n/ because the co-articulatory transition from a tongue-tip contact to tongue-dorsum contact may be difficult and confusing until the placement is well established. When production is easier, words with tongue-tip sounds may be added, such as "running, tongue."

Velar Plosives

Nasal occlusion imposed during production of the sustained velar nasal will elicit a velar plosive /g/. The release should initially be over-aspirated, using the /h/ as described above. The child should produce repetitions of /iŋgi-iŋgi-iŋgi/ producing /ŋg/ in the medial position. The vowel /i/ is a useful facilitator because, as a high vowel, it elicits elevation of the tongue dorsum. When the clinician occludes the nares, a velar plosive /g/ will emerge. Other useful stimulus words for pairing the nasal /ŋ/ with a velar plosive are "uncle, hanger, anger, monkey, bank, dunk." The next step is to produce this sequence followed by the target syllable /gi/, that is, the sequence to be produced is /iŋgi-gi/." This should be produced correctly five consecutive times to establish production in the initial word position. The vowel can be changed to be sure the child can produce the sequence with both front and back vowels. The procedure for phasing out use of the nasal occlusion and nasal phoneme as a facilitator is the same as described above. The velar plosives differ from the other sounds in that the voiced /g/ usually seems easier than voiceless /k/. Nasal /ŋ/ and plosive /g/ can be used to facilitate production of voiceless /k/ with the cue to "make the sound very windy." To elicit production in the medial position, the child can precede initial /k/ words with "a," as in "a key, a cake, a car." Words that can be produced correctly at this stage include: kay, key, cookie, cake, make, "q," come, came, go, girl, gone, gum, game, gang. As noted above, words containing /n, t, d/ should not be introduced until /k, g, ŋ/ are well established in repetition at the word level, usually one or two sessions after their introduction. Then, words may include: tongue, cat, goat, tag, got, king, queen.

Back Sounds, Low Pressure-Retroflex

If developmentally appropriate, /r/ may be introduced after the velars because it is another posterior sound. In fact, the blends "gr" and "kr" are among the most effective facilitators for /r/. Instructions for /ɝ/(er) production, often the most stimulable r-context, are to "close the back teeth, smile, and curl the tongue-tip back to tickle your throat with your tongue." The most common errors on /r/, substitution of /w/ or /v/, result from an attempt to produce the sound using the lips rather than the tongue. The patient should be told that /r/ is a "tongue sound" and not a "lip sound." The instructions provided prevent use of the lips. Closing the teeth provides jaw stability and smiling retracts the lips and eliminates their use for the sound. When the child is prevented from moving other articulators, they use tongue. As was just said, pairing /r/ with a velar consonant facilitates tongue retraction and is often helpful. Vowels requiring lip rounding should be avoided when /r/ is first introduced because their presence either before or after the /r/ will result in co-articulatory lip rounding during the /r/. These vowel contexts should be introduced when /r/ production in other vowel contexts is stable. Examples of good initial contexts are "Greek, creek, gray, cry, crayon." When /r/ is produced correctly at the word level in velar blends, tongue-tip consonant blends (tr, dr) can be introduced. This releases the tongue-backing facilitator but maintains the lip retraction, making these blends easier than those including bilabial sounds, which should be introduced last.

Velar sounds were described following the bilabial and lingua-alveolar plosives because of the similarity in usual error (glottal stop) and elicitation techniques. The principle of moving from front sounds to back sounds has been emphasized. The clinician must judge, on a case by case basis, if velars should be introduced in this sequence or held even longer and trained following front fricatives. This is considered in Chapter 7.

Front Sounds, High Pressure

Labiodental Fricatives

The first fricatives to be introduced are usually /f/ and /v/ because they are anterior, visible, and the earliest developing fricatives. The most common compensatory error produced for these sounds is a pharyngeal fricative, although some children substitute nasal snorting or even glottal stops. Initial production should be with the nares occluded. Production is effected by using the maxillary teeth to lightly bite the inner edge of the lower lip. A common error is to tell the child to "bite the lip," which often results in complete in-turning of the lower lip. The contact between the teeth and lower lip should be tight enough to create friction, but not so hard as to make tooth marks, which we have seen happen. Production begins with the nares occluded by the clinician, labiodental contact in place followed by a "Big HHHHHHHH." This should be repeated until there are five consecutive correct productions of /f/ sustained for at least 5 seconds. The child should then be told that the clinician may let go of the nose, but the child is to keep making the wind come out of the mouth and not stop making the sound. Production of the next sequence begins with the nares occluded. After initiation of correct /f/ production, the clinician should release the nares for 1 second, then occlude them for the remainder of the sustained /f/. Specific verbal reinforcement should be given, such as "Good! You kept the wind coming!" and another repetition should be initiated until there are five consecutive correct productions starting and ending with the nares occluded. The next step is to begin with nares occluded, then release and sustain oral /f/ for the remainder of the 5 seconds, without re-occluding the nares. After five consecutive correct productions, the child should begin with the nares open, but with the clinician's fingers or a nose clip in ready position on either side of the nares. The child should begin the production with the nares opened, and after 2 seconds, they should be closed. This provides evidence that the air stream was directed orally, rather than nasally. This should be repeated until there are five consecutive correct productions, followed by five productions of sustained /f/ with the nose open. The clinician should then move immediately to /f/ + vowel syllables. The syllables should be produced with a prolonged /ffffffff/ for emphasis. Syllables may include: fay, fee, figh, fo, foo. Little children enjoy pretending to be the Giant in "Jack and the Beanstalk," and going home practicing, "Fee, Figh, Fo, Fum."

The next step is to introduce medial and final position /f/. If the child has difficulty repeating nonsense syllables with the nose open, the procedure used to establish initial position /f/ may be repeated with medial and final /f/. Practice words to be added to the repertoire of correctly produced words include, "food, finger, farmer, family, before, feel, four, fat, fight, foot, feet, feed, fed, fit, fair, fear, fire, fur, far, fun, funny, fell, fall, full, puff, puffy, muff, Muffy, taffy, Rafi, Daffy, calf, elephant, forget, beautiful, wonderful."

To elicit /v/, the child should sustain /f/ while "buzzing" or "humming." This will add voicing to the /f/, resulting in production of sustained /v/. If this proves difficult with the nose open, the steps for eliciting /f/ should be repeated with voicing added to shape the /f/ into /v/. The corpus of words may then be expanded to include: five, vine, very, every, everyone, dive, diving, hive, vote, view, over, even, favor, whatever, give, gave, have, move, above, believe, even, evening, wave.

One of the most useful /v/ words is "have." Short, structured phrases are used to establish production of target sounds after criteria is reached at the word level. The entire repertoire of words and pictures can be paired with this word in the phrase "I have _____."

The child is able to review production of previously learned sounds using this phrase, while moving to the syllable and word level for the next group of sounds.

(Tongue-tip) Interdental Fricatives

Voiceless and voiced /θ/ and /ð/ are usually the next fricative sounds introduced because they are anterior and visible. Once established, they can also be used as effective facilitators for teaching /s/ and /z/. The voiceless /θ/ is introduced first, using the sequence described for /f/. The only difference is that upper and lower teeth are in contact with the tongue tip. The instruction, "Bite your tongue" may be used, but care must be taken that the child does not overclose on the tongue causing discomfort, and that the child does not attempt to protrude the dorsum of the tongue. If the child learns overextension of the tongue, it may be difficult for them to make rapid co-articulatory movements. In fact, the sound is not produced with the tongue fully extended between the teeth. It is produced with the tip of the tongue placed gently between the maxillary and mandibular teeth. After production of sustained voiceless /θ/ in isolation with the nose closed and opened is established as described above, the sound should be produced in syllables with all vowels: thay, thee, thigh, tho, thu, thæ, theh, thih, thoh, thuh. Voiceless /θ/ can be used as a facilitator to teach voiced /ð/ using the same procedure as was described in shaping /f/ to /v/. Words that can now be added to the child's corpus of correctly produced words include: thumb, thing, mouth, moth, mother, father, thick, thin, three, through, anything, nothing, everything, tooth, both, path, they, there, that, the, without, them, then, another, together, weather, with.

Lingua-alveolar Sibilants

Logically, the next sounds to introduce are sibilants /s/ and /z/. There are several ways to teach these sounds. One way is to use /θ/ as a facilitator. The child should be told to produce /θ/ with the teeth closed. The first productions should be done with nasal occlusion as described in the previous sections, especially if the error was nasal snorting. This almost always results in production of /s/. If the sound is still closer to /θ/ than /s/, the child should be told to pull the tongue inside a bit more, to the spot "where the teeth enter the gum." This usually results in sibilant production. If the individual overcompensates for the tongue position and produces /ʃ/, that sound may be targeted prior to /s/. If not, /ʃ/ should be introduced following /s/ and /z/.

Tongue-tip /t/ may also be used as facilitator for /s/. The individual should be asked to sustain a loud /t/, often resulting in /s/. Another way to establish /s/ is to use a coffee stirrer, inserted lengthwise along the surface of the tongue, creating a central groove in the tongue. The individual should then produce a strong, sustained /t/ sound. The /t/ can be used as a phonetic facilitator in some words, often eliciting the first /s/ productions in the final word position. For example, if the child is asked to say "cat" and sustain the /t/, the result will be production of "cats." The sound should then be repeated, as in "cats—ssssss." Each stimulus word or word pair should be repeated until there are five consecutive correct productions. Nasal occlusion should be used as necessary, following the procedure described previously. The /s/ can then be used as a facilitator to elicit /z/ by adding voicing. This should be done during a single sustained production: sssssssszzzzzzzzz. After pairing the /s/ and /z/ with each vowel, words may be added to the child's list. If the child's error was any type of nasal fricative, it is best to introduce fully oral words which are words excluding nasal sounds, such as sun, some, same. Words containing sibilants and nasals should only be introduced after correct production of fully oral words with the nose open is established. Words that can be added are: say, sea, sigh, sew, Sue, saw, suit, side, south, sit, sat, seat, seed, say, bus, pass, yes, city, sick, silver, sister, salt, save, safe, kiss, yes, ice, house, voice, base. When production of voiced /z/ is established in z + vowel syllables, words may include: zoo, zebra, these, is, as, because, rose, use, his, was, please, rise, peas, bees, and plural forms of other nouns previously learned.

SIBILANT BLENDS. Depending on the developmental level of the child, it may be appropriate to introduce s-blends. Oral blends should be introduced first, and sm- and sn- blends should be introduced last, progressing from easiest to most difficult transitions. The nasal blends should be taught only after adequate tongue control and oral airflow for production of the oral blends has been demonstrated. This does not mean that nasal emission or nasal turbulence will be absent, especially if there is still a palatal fistula or VPI. It means that nasal snorting (nasal fricatives) will be absent and that production will be correct with the nares occluded.

Lingua-palatal Fricative

The /s/ can be used as a facilitator to teach /ʃ/ (sh) by retracting the tongue into the middle of the mouth. It is helpful to start with /s/ and pull the tongue in while sustaining the "Big HHHH" so that the sound transitions from /s/ to /ʃ/ for several trials. The use of nasal occlusion and release may be applied as described in the previous sections, although it is often no longer necessary at this stage of treatment. Like /r/, distorted /ʃ/ is often accompanied by lip protrusion and rounding. The patient should be told that /ʃ/ is a tongue sound, not a lip sound. It should be taught with the lips retracted, avoiding lip-round vowels in the initially introduced contexts. Use of a mirror is important so that the patient can see that he or she is "being a ventriloquist" and not releasing the lip retraction. Once the sound is stable in these contexts, the lip-round vowels can be added.

Affricates

The transition from /ʃ/ to affricates /tʃ/ and /dʒ/ is simple. If the child is old enough to read, the first stimuli should be words containing t + sh/ch or d + j so there is a clear graphic (visual) cue to produce both the plosive and fricative, such as "match, catch, patch, badge, edge." The words can be written "matsh, catsh," and so on to make the point. For a younger child, the affricates can be elicited by telling them to make the "sh" stronger, or to "make a sneezing sound." The affricates can usually be elicited by imitation of the adult model, using /ʃ/ as the facilitator. All phonemes have been introduced at this point, so there are no phonetic restrictions on target words. If the child has some difficulty with certain words, the phonetic context should be analyzed and a determination can be made as to whether or not a particular group of words should be introduced at a later time. For example, if the child continues to have difficulty with oral-nasal contrasts, words such as "bunch, lunch" should be introduced at a later time, when production of "ch" is more stable.

STRENGTH OF ARTICULATORY CONTACTS

The use of strong articulatory contacts should be encouraged, especially if there is weak intraoral pressure. The use of light articulatory contacts to decrease the perception of hypernasality has been recommended (McWilliams et al., 1990; Van Demark & Hardin, 1990). Although it is true that increasing the strength of articulatory contacts may result in an increase in nasal turbulence, it has the benefit of improved speech intelligibility. It may also be associated with improved velopharyngeal motion (Hoch et al., 1986; Golding-Kushner, 1989). Increasing strength of articulatory contacts means using the lips and tongue in a more forceful way to produce sounds. For example, the lips should be pressed together for /p/, not just made to come into contact with each other. Increasing the strength of articulatory contacts should not be confused with doing exercises to increase lip/tongue strength or with increasing vocal intensity. Exercises to increase lip, tongue, or jaw strength are inappropriate because there is not a proven relationship between strength of individual oral structures and accuracy of articulation. This is discussed in detail in Chapter 9.

TREATMENT OF HYPERNASALITY WITHOUT COMPENSATORY ARTICULATION

Hypernasality is an abnormal resonance characteristic that is usually a consequence of VPI. As discussed in Chapter 3, elimination of abnormal compensatory errors often results in an increase in velopharyngeal motion which may or may not be accompanied by a decrease in hypernasality. It must be emphasized that the goal of articulation therapy is to eliminate the compensatory errors. The goal is not to change VP motion or to reduce hypernasality. That is simply a benefit that is sometimes observed.

What about individuals who are hypernasal and have developmental or other articulation errors? What about individuals who are hypernasal but, aside from reduced intraoral pressure, have normal articulation? It bears repeating that hypernasality is a perceptual phenomenon, not a physiological event. Before deciding to attempt speech therapy to decrease hypernasality, the patient *must* undergo testing to visualize velopharyngeal closure during unimpeded, connected speech. As stated earlier, this can only be accomplished using nasopharyngoscopy and multiview videofluoroscopy. There are several possible results of these evaluations for children without compensatory errors:

1. If VPI is *consistently* present, speech therapy will **not** be of benefit. Physical management of VPI should be considered.
2. If VPI is *inconsistently* present, careful phonetic analysis should be done to determine when VP closure is achieved and when it is not.
   a. Variations in VP closure may be phonetically based. A speech therapy procedure would be to use phonemes accompanied by good closure to facilitate improved production of other phonemes.
   b. Variations in VP closure may be related to timing of VP closure. That is, closure may be achieved late or released early during

transitions between nasal and non-nasal phonemes or during transitions between voiceless and voiced phonemes. These transitions can be made a speech therapy goal. Visual feedback of closure is very helpful for this. Therefore, treatment using endoscopic biofeedback might be useful.

c. Variations in VP closure might be related to strength of articulatory contacts and speech effort made by the speaker. If so, increasing the strength of articulatory contacts and speech effort would be an appropriate therapy target.

The key is to perform a careful analysis of the endoscopic examination to determine the speech characteristics that accompany variations in VP closure. The speech features that occur during good closure can be used to facilitate improvement in other phonemes by pairing them together. This type of treatment should be considered diagnostic, and reevaluation after 2 months of intensive treatment should be done to determine if therapy should continue or not.

It is obvious that most SLPs working in the community do not have endoscopes. However, it is important that patients with hypernasality be referred for appropriate evaluation prior to undertaking speech therapy. The reason for this should be obvious. If VPI is consistent, therapy is not appropriate. If VPI is inconsistent, there is no way to select appropriate therapy techniques without the information derived from direct testing. In summary, speech therapy for VPI is limited to those situations in which nasopharyngoscopy or multiview videofluoroscopy clearly show a predictable pattern of variability associated with speech activity.

USING TECHNOLOGY IN TREATMENT

Some clinicians have access to tools that take advantage of advances in technology. It is essential to differentiate the *tools* from *techniques*. Example of tools are palatometers, nasometers, computer speech programs, and pressure-flow apparatus. Lower technology tools include nasal emission mirrors, See-Scape™, and stethescopes. These tools are not intended to provide direct information about the configuration of velopharyngeal closure, although inferences about closure are often erroneously made. The output of the nasometer, for example, is a ratio of oral:nasal resonance. It is not designed to look at velopharyngeal closure or articulation. Some clinicians are comfortable using these tools and, within their limits, they may be useful therapy tools for some patients. Any tool can be used to facilitate therapy, as long as its use is not in conflict with the therapy techniques and principles that work. It is important to avoid reliance on tools that are clinician, room, or time dependent because they foster dependence and interfere with progress when they are not available for a particular session. Dependency on a tool also hinders movement to higher levels of treatment and carry over. Consideration should be given to the fact that similar "objective" feedback ("Yes, nasal air-flow is present") may be obtained from more than one tool, such as from pressure-flow and a stethescope.

AVOIDING THE PITFALLS

Although we have mentioned this already, the risk of inadvertently establishing a pattern of co-produced glottal stops or intrusive glottal stops or pharyngeal fricatives bears special mention. Some patients learn correct production of sounds but continue to insert the error sound with, or immediately after, the correct production. This may be avoided by a strong emphasis on airflow direction and by avoiding an exclusive focus on lip and tongue placement. The speech pathologist should cue and reinforce airflow manner as well as the place at which the airstream is modified. For example, it is better to elicit the sound /b/ with an instruction such as "stop the air with your lips," than with a statement such as "close your lips." Statements used to elicit and reinforce sound production must be *specific* and state both which articulators to use and what the articulators are doing to the air. The clinician and individual should be constantly aware that the reason for using the articulators is to do something to the outgoing airstream. It is the airstream that is primary. Without air, there is no speech.

HYPONASALITY

Hyponasality often occurs following pharyngeal flap surgery and improves in time, usually within 6 months. Individuals with chronic hyponasality of unknown origin should be examined by an otolaryngologist to determine the cause. Enlarged adenoids, deviated nasal septum, and allergic rhinitis are common causes, and medical treatment is often possible. If it is not, the perception of hyponasality may be reduced by increasing the duration of nasal phonemes.

CHAPTER

7

After the Sound: Selection and Sequencing of Target Sounds and from Sounds to Conversation

Establishing correct production of consonants in syllables and simple words without compensatory errors is a significant task. Of course, the ultimate goal is to transfer, or generalize, correct production to conversational speech with automaticity. This goal must be approached in a methodical way. Several parameters of treatment must be considered, including the sequence of target sounds, when to introduce additional sounds, phonetic complexity of target words, how to move up and across levels of therapy from syllables through conversation, linguistic complexity of the therapy task, and the therapeutic awareness of the individual's conversational partner.

SEQUENCING OF TARGET SOUNDS

Target sounds must be selected and sequenced for therapy. The developmental sequence of articulatory mastery is one consideration. Sounds should be maturationally appropriate for the child. In general, treatment begins with /h/ and then proceeds from front sounds to back sounds. Within these parameters, the choice of specific phonemes should be based on results of stimulability testing and begin with sounds most easily produced by the individual. A typical sequence for the introduction of sounds is found in Table 7–1.

This list is based on the principle to begin with /h/ to break the glottal stop pattern, then concentrate on front sounds. Voiceless sounds are usually easier than voiced sounds. Therefore, in most cases, voiceless sounds are introduced before their voiced cognates. The goal is to move articulation forward. A simple mantra to share with the patient is "back is bad, front is fine." The information in Table 7–1 is a general guide and must be adapted for each patient based on factors, including maturational age, linguistic level of development, and stimulability test results. For example, some children progress more quickly when "th" is introduced before /t, d/. The tongue tip placement is even more forward for "th" and provides a greater contrast to the undesireable tongue backing pattern being broken. Regardless of which is introduced first, the sounds /θ, ð, t, d/ provide mutual reinforcement for forward tongue-tip placement in spite of their difference in air-flow management (fricative vs. plosive).

The degree to which an error deviates from the target should also be considered. Some individuals do well when the target sound has multiple features in contrast with the error. For example, fricative /f/ and a glottal stop differ in place and manner of articulation, two features. For others, the initial targets should involve changing a single

TABLE 7–1. *Sample Therapeutic Sequence for Phonemes*

Group Number	Place of Articulation	Phonemes
1	laryngeal	/h/ (aspirate)
2	bilabial	/w, m, p, b/
3	labiodental	/f, v/
4	tongue-tip	/n, t, d/
5	tongue-tip	/θ, ð/
6	tongue-tip	/s, z/
7	velar	/ŋ, g, k/
8	mid-palatal	/ʃ/
9	mid-palatal	/tʃ, dʒ/

feature, namely, place of articulation. When glottal stops are substituted for oral stops, the error is in place of articulation (a single feature). The type of error is backing. In most cases, it is recommended to focus on a shift in one feature of sound production first, then move to sounds with two features in error or to a sound that is only one feature removed from the last sound learned.

Low pressure sounds that were not listed in Table 7–1, including /r, l/ should be introduced when developmentally appropriate. As indicated in the previous chapter, it is often helpful to group /r/ with the velar sounds. Similarly, /l/ would be logically grouped with the other tongue-tip sounds /n, t, d/. If a child is in treatment to eliminate abnormal compensatory errors prior to surgery, the pressure sounds need to take priority and the low-pressure sounds, which are less likely to be produced as glottal stops and more likely to be distorted by developmental errors, should be held until the glottal stops are eliminated.

Phonetic "Chunking" versus Phonological Categorization

In Table 7–1, sounds listed together are generally introduced in the order listed. However, they can be approached as a group if the child is able to handle several sounds at once. This type of goal "chunking" may, at first glance, seem similar to a phonological approach to the disorder. However, the chunking is according to phonetic parameters that are the desired features of the target sounds, especially place and manner of articulation. In contrast, phonological approach groups sounds according to the common error. For a child with a pervasive glottal stop speech disorder, phonetic chunking has the advantage often attributed to phonological approaches of speeding treatment by training several phonemes at once. At the same time, it avoids a negative aspect of phonological treatment by grouping the phonemes more specifically and according to the goal. That is, the goal might be "to establish correct production of bilabial plosives," rather than "to eliminate glottal replacements." While the ultimate objective is, obviously, to eliminate compensatory errors, phonetic sound chunking keeps the focus on establishing production of groups of sounds that have similar physiological features and on correct production of the specific sounds, not on eliminating a "process." The undesirable behavior must be replaced with the correct physiological events. Read carefully—this difference goes beyond mere semantics.

The criterion levels listed in the sections that follow apply to individual sound targets as well as to sound groups. The criteria provide guidelines for moving between levels of complexity from syllable to conversation for individual sounds. There is not a particular criterion that must be met on a sound before another sound can be introduced. That decision must be based on the patient's ability to handle two or more sounds at one time. They are usually able to handle more as therapy progresses. As a result, most patients begin treatment by working on one sound, usually /h/, and then increase the number of targets as they become more accustomed to therapy and the therapeutic process.

STIMULABILITY TESTING

Stimulability testing, or probing to determine the most effective procedure for eliciting correct production of an error sound, should be done at the time of speech evaluation. If for some reason it has not been done at that time, it should be accomplished at the first clinical visit. When stimulability testing is done properly, correct production of at least some error sounds will be elicited at that first visit. True stimulability testing goes beyond a request to repeat a sound or word heard. It demands the application of therapy principles and procedures in microcosm. During stimulability testing, various types of cues are used to elicit production of a sound. These cues may be auditory, visual, phonetic, verbal, manual, and/or tactile. One or two attempts to elicit the sound should be tried using those types of cues and may be used in combination.

The most common type of elicitation uses *auditory* cues. The clinician produces a model and the patient repeats a sound or word produced. Repetition is sometimes elicited directly ("Say what I say"). At other times, especially with young children, it may be elicited indirectly during play activities in which the child spontaneously repeats the clinician's model within a relevant linguistic context. For example, if the clinician says "My owl said 'whoooooo,'" the child holding another toy owl is likely to say 'whoooooo.'"

There are several types of *visual* cues. Visual placement cues are provided when the patient watches the therapist's use of articulators directly or in a mirror (Figure 7–1). This should also be used in conjunction with visual airflow cues to avoid co-production of glottal stops. Visual airflow cues may be provided to the patient using a mirror, feather, or cotton ball held near the mouth to provide visual feedback of oral airflow (Figures 7–2 and 7–3). *This is not a blowing exercise.* It is important to be sure that the feedback tool (cotton ball, tissue, etc.) is held in a position that will prevent its response to nasal air flow that is obligatory, such as nasal emission, or that would inadvertently reinforce incorrect speech responses, such as nasal snorting. Visual placement cues can also be provided by the clinician mouthing the word while the individual produces it. Watching the clinician and then producing the word provides visual cues that the individual must hold in memory; mouthing as the child speaks provides a type of "on-line" support. This type of cueing is especially useful when the child is making his or her first attempts at delayed repetition (the clinician says a word, the individual repeats it five times in sequence such that four of the repetitions are not immediately preceded by the clinicians model).

Another type of cue is *phonetic*. Using phonetic cues, a sound that is produced correctly by the individual is used as a facilitator to elicit another. For example, if the individual can produce voiceless "th" correctly, they can be asked to produce and sustain /θ/ with the teeth closed, which will result in production of /s/. Another example is whispering a correctly produced voiced sound, such as /v/ or /dɑ/ to elicit the voiceless cognate /f/ or /tɑ/.

The next type of cue is *verbal*. This is one of the simplest but most misused cues. With this type of cue, the clinician provides specific instructions for articulation placement and manner of airstream management. An example of verbal cuing for /s/ is "Put your tongue behind your teeth and make the air come out your mouth." A common error by clinicians is to omit the verbal instructions for airflow management in addition to the instructions for articulation placement. This may result

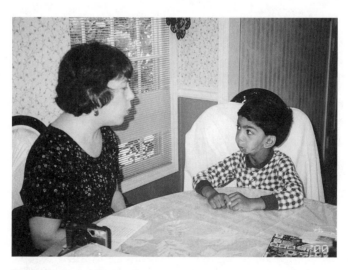

FIGURE 7–1. Visual placement cues for sound production: The patient watches and imitates how the clinician moves her articulators.

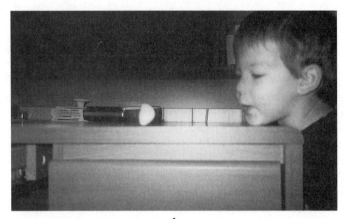

A

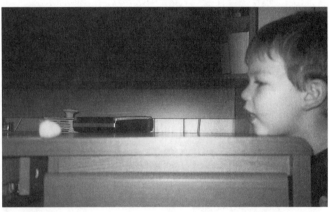

B

FIGURE 7–2. Visual cues: Visual airflow cues may be provided using a cotton ball that becomes displaced by oral airflow during correct oral production of pressure consonants, in this case, /pɑ/. The cotton ball becomes slightly displaced at the initial /p/ release (**A**), and moves farther as the aspiraton is released (**B**). *This is not a blowing exercise.*

in lip and tongue movement and placement and the appearance of improvement. However, when the airflow cues are omitted, compensatory errors may persist or be co-produced and be inadvertently reinforced.

Manual cues or assistance are provided when the therapist manipulates the lips, tongue, or nose of the patient. Examples are gently closing the individual's nares to force *oral* air emission during fricative and

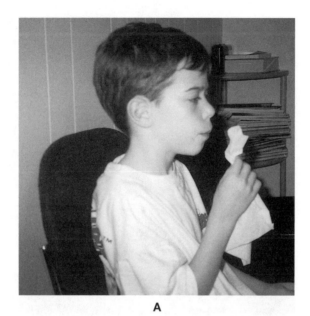

A

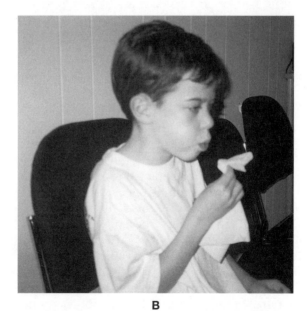

B

FIGURE 7–3. Visual cues: Visual airflow cues and feedback can also be obtained using a tissue held just below the mouth. Here, the child says, "Pooh" (**A**) with good lip closure for the initial /p/ and (**B**) release of aspiration with lip rounding for /u/. *This is not a blowing exercise.*

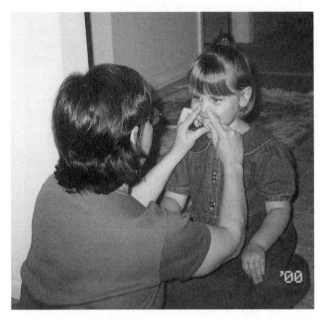

FIGURE 7–4. Manual cues: Manual assistance can be used to facilitate establishment of oral airflow, especially during production of sibilants and fricatives. Here, the clinician occludes the nares to establish oral airflow and simultaneously provides gentle manipulation of the mandible and lower lip to teach correct placement of the articulators for /f/. Training in correct sound production should always include cues for both placement of articulators *and* airflow management.

sibilant production (Figure 7–4), and using a tongue depressor to hold the tongue tip down during training of velar sounds (Figure 7–5).

Another type of cue is *tactile*. Touch may be used to provide the patient with feedback about some aspect of production, such as feeling a puff of air from the mouth on the hand (Figure 7–6), or feeling labial pressure during production of bilabial sounds on a finger (Figure 7–7).

Stimulability testing is critical for several reasons. First, it immediately establishes a recognition of the ability to speak correctly for the child and parents. Second, results of stimulability testing are an important factor in establishing the sequence of sounds to target in therapy. In addition, the results provide insight to the clinician about what procedures may be most effective with a particular patient. Results of stimulability testing should not be considered final, and all conclusions

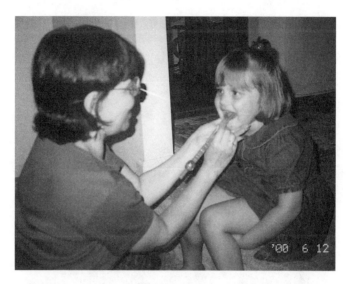

FIGURE 7–5. Manual cues: The clinician provides manual cues to elicit production of velar consonants by using a plastic straw to hold the tongue tip down.

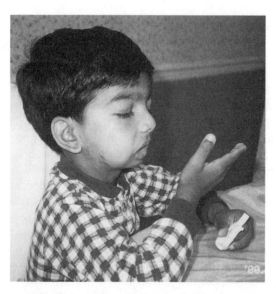

FIGURE 7–6. Tactile cues: Tactile cues might include feeling the release of a puff of air during production of plosive /p/ on the hand.

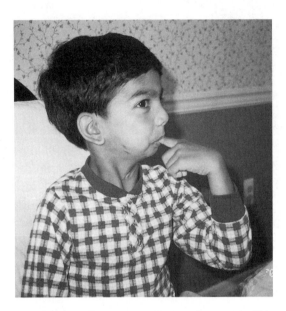

FIGURE 7–7. Tactile cues: Using a finger to feel bilabial closure and oral air pressure during production of /p/.

should be considered provisional. What seems to be easiest for an individual when they are first starting treatment may not be easiest at a different stage.

School speech clinicians may face a dilemma regarding stimulability testing. In some school districts, one criteria for *exclusion* from school services is a demonstrated ability to produce the sound. The law in a particular state or district may indicate that a child is eligible for speech services at school only if they have not demonstrated the ability to produce the error sounds correctly. In this situation, the law unfortunately and erroneously assumes that if a child can produce a sound correctly "so easily" at the time of the evaluation, they will learn to produce it on their own and do not require intervention. In other words, the law writers in this situation believe the therapy process must be long and difficult. They believe that, if it is so easy for the child to produce the sound correctly, the disorder cannot be so bad and the child must not need professional services. When this situation exists, the clinician may make the decision to omit stimulability testing or only include superficial sound stimulation at the time of evaluation and reserve true stimulability testing for the first therapy session. A major disadvantage to this approach is that goals will be established for the IEP without benefit of stimulability testing results.

LEVELS OF THERAPY:
WHERE TO BEGIN AND WHERE TO GO

In the previous chapter, techniques to elicit production of sounds and to eliminate production of compensatory errors were described. In this section, we will consider the contexts in which those sounds are presented. Levels of therapy include production of the sound in isolation, syllables, words, phrases, sentences, and conversation. Articulation tests generally elicit production of sounds in words or sentences. Sounds are elicited in isolation, syllables and/or words during stimulability testing. Treatment should begin at the lowest level at which success is achieved. This level will vary from individual to individual. In fact, for a single patient, the level may vary from one sound to the next. Some individuals begin treatment for a particular sound at the word level, some at the syllable level, some in isolation. Contexts for each level will be described.

Criterion Levels

Beginning at the word level, the criterion for moving to the next level of treatment is 90% accuracy *and* production of a minimum of 100 correct responses during two consecutive sessions. The 90% accuracy level is recommended in order to ensure that complete mastery of production at each level is achieved before moving on. Lower levels of accuracy are accepted by some clinicians, but this does not provide the same foundation for success as the patient moves from level to level. When the next linguistic level is introduced, a minimum of 30% accuracy in repetition should be achieved. If it is not, the individual should return to the previous level for a few minutes, until there are five consecutive correct productions. Then a stimulus at the new level can be re-introduced in a phonetically matched sequence. As an example, a child having difficulty moving from /h/ in syllables to words could repeat "ho-ho-ho-home." The goal would then be five consecutive correct repetitions of the sequence, at which time an attempt could be made to repeat the word "home" without the preliminary syllable repetition. The clinician can mouth the word as the client makes his attempt to provide visual cueing for completion of the word.

It must be emphasized that a central focus of all sound production is proper airflow direction. Whenever necessary, liberal use of nasal occlusion should be used. The patient should always be reminded to push air out of the mouth. After each sequence of five productions with the nares occluded, the stimulus should be produced with the nares open, then occluded. When the nostrils are open the clinician must be careful to differentiate between obligatory nasal emission and compensatory nasal snorting. This can be monitored by applying nasal occlusion mid-production of the target sound within the word. Obviously, the clinician must use precise timing to apply this type of nasal occlusion so that it will serve a monitoring function.

Isolation

Continuant sounds can be produced in isolation, but plosives cannot. Therefore, this level of complexity applies to vowels, semivowels, nasals, and fricatives. The sound is elicited first by imitation of the clinician's model. If this is not effective on two or three repetitions, other types of cueing, described in the section on stimulability testing, should be used. A verbal description of production should always be given as well. If the sound was not imitated correctly, the description serves as a production cue. If the sound *was* imitated correctly, the description acts as positive, specific reinforcement. The verbal description must include both the articulatory placement information *and* the airflow information. For example, if the target sound is /f/, an appropriate statement is, "Good! You bit your lip a little and pushed the air out your mouth." The first set of repetitions should be done with the clinician modeling the sound for each of five repetitions. The next sequence should be the clinician's model followed by five consecutive productions by the individual (delayed repetition). The third sequence in isolation is for the clinician to cue by saying "more" or "again." Most individuals complete the isolation level of a particular sound in 5 minutes or less. The sound should be produced in isolation until there are five consecutive correct productions at each of the three levels, at which time syllables may be introduced.

Syllables

All sounds can be produced at the syllable level. The child should repeat syllables produced by the clinician. Consonant-vowel (CV) syllables are introduced first most of the time because they are usually easier than VC syllables and, as pointed out previously, VC syllables actually have a glottal onset. Therefore, VC syllables should be used judiciously at this early stage of therapy. Although it does result in production of some nonsense syllables, the "V" should be replaced by every vowel and diphthong for practice. This enables the individual to produce the sound with front, back, high, and low vowels. Physiologically, this provides training and experience in combining correct articulatory placement for the target sound while transitioning to or from varying tongue and lip positions. Special note should be made of specific contexts that are difficult for the individual, and those may be isolated for additional practice. The child should repeat each CV combination after the clinician five times. The combination should then be produced five times after a single model, and then five consecutive times without a model. These sequences should be continued until there are five consecutive correct responses for each CV and /h/ plus VC context. After the criterion level is reached, the meaningful CV and /h/VC syllables should be selected for home and additional clinical practice. For younger children, the syllables can be represented in pictures. For readers, they may be written into the speech book for home practice. Meaningful syllables form the core of first words correctly produced with the target sound. When the patient can repeat the monosyllabic words correctly five consecutive times, the individual should move to naming. The individual should name target pictures or read target words until 90% accuracy is achieved at two consecutive visits. A minimum of 100 correct productions should occur at each visit. Therefore, achieving 90% accuracy requires 112 attempts. When this criterion level has been reached, the word level may be introduced for that sound.

Strength of Articulatory Contacts

At all levels of therapy, production of strong articulatory contacts should be stressed. This should not be confused with strength of the articulators. As previously stated, the lips and tongue of speakers with "cleft palate speech" are not weak. They simply are not used. When individuals begin to use the articulators to produce sounds being taught, they may be inclined to make light contact at points of articulation. Earlier treatment programs even advocated teaching light contacts. It is our experience that encouraging speakers to use strong articulation contacts enhances speech intelligibility by increasing the precision of articulation. This should be included as a goal from the introduction of sounds through the conversational level of treatment.

Words

The first words introduced usually have CVC construction, building logically on the syllable level and providing an easy physiological transition between levels. Using a few trials of each, the clinician should determine if the individual can say a particular sound with greater accuracy in the initial or final word position and begin with that structure. Some sounds, such as velar nasal /ŋ/ and velar plosives /k, g/ may be easiest in the medial position of words and should be introduced in VCV nonsense words.

As discussed previously, target words should be selected that can be correctly produced by the individual. Therefore, the final "C" in the CVC sequence will depend on the child's repertoire. As proficiency in production of the target sound in the initial word position increases, words with increased syllabic complexity may be presented.

Words should be presented in repetition until there are at least 100 correct responses with 90% accuracy during two consecutive sessions. When this level of accuracy is achieved in repetition, word naming may be introduced. The first words presented at the naming level should be the same as the ones that were used during the repetition task. Naming is slightly more complex than repetition because the child must produce the target without the clinician's model. However, using the same words as were used during repetition increases the likelihood of success. If a 30% level of accuracy is not achieved on the first ten trials, the words should be produced in repetition for an additional 5 to 10 minutes, and naming may be tried again. If the level of accuracy is at least 30%, naming may continue, but when any word is produced incorrectly, the clinician should provide a model and the child should repeat it, then the next word can be named. Providing a verbal cue to remind the child how to produce the sound prior to each production also maximizes success. Verbal production cues may be faded out as accuracy in naming increases and as the child exhibits increased confidence in his or her ability to produce the sound.

The procedure for guiding a child from accurate production in syllables to production in conversation involves a series of linguistic and physiologic transitions from simple to complex, supported by cueing that decreases from maximum to none. The next transitional phase at the word level is to elicit production of single words without the clinician's model and without the visual cue provided by pictures. One method of doing this is for the clinician to ask questions to elicit specific target words that the child must answer using a word containing the target sound. The questions should be asked according to the child's interests, not the clinician's. It is important to keep questions, monologues, dialogues, and other therapy topics within a linguistically meaningful context. For example, talking about their everyday activities (bath, meals, bedtime) is appropriate for young children, but may be boring for older children, who may be more interested in sports or the latest CD.

Word Combinations and Phrases

Once the child is able to say some single words, two words can be combined to establish production in slightly longer sequences. Using the target sound /h/, the child might "greet" every picture in his speech book using the word paired with "hi" ("Hi, home; Hi, hole; Hi, him"). For target sound /m/, the word combination could use "my" ("My mommy; My man; My moo"). In addition to reinforcing correct production in a rudimentary phrase, this type of structure elicits sounds in the medial position of a phonetic sequence, providing additional practice. This level of treatment should be introduced in the same way as previous levels, using repetition first, then fading out the clinician's model. The same criterion levels apply.

Carrier phrases provide an excellent transition to the sentence level because the target word is phonetically embedded in a sentence, but the child can focus on production without also having to engage in the linguistic task of generating a sentence. The same carrier phrase can be used to describe each picture. Examples of carrier phrases are "I have _____," "I want _____," "I see _____," and "A _____ here." The choice of carrier phrase is determined by the sounds that the child can say correctly because the principle of completely correct production during therapy tasks continues to apply.

Reinforcement for correct production of the carrier phrase and target words often takes the form of a turn at a game. Once the child achieves the criterion level for use of the carrier phrase, select carrier phrases can be used in games themselves. This is a more complex level of production because the child's attention is divided between articulating the sounds and phrases and playing the game, thus demanding slightly more automaticity of speech. Games that require talking are excellent for this level of treatment, including card games like Go Fish! War, and Memory, and board games like Guess Who? and Battleship. The carrier phrases should be created as appropriate to the game and phonetic competence, and different carrier phrases may be used for the same game at different times. This is described in detail in Chapter 8.

Sentences

The next level of linguistic and phonetic complexity is production of target words in sentences. Because of the importance of complete articulatory accuracy within therapeutic tasks, sentences cannot be introduced until the child is able to produce enough sounds at the carrier phrase level to generate sentences. Because sentences will often be introduced before all sounds are correct in phrases, the first sentences should be generated by the clinician. In this way, sounds that are not yet produced correctly can be excluded from the sentence. Once criterion is reached for all phonemes in phrases, novel sentences can be generated by the patient. This does not mean that the child cannot produce sentences until criterion is met for all sounds in phrases. It means that production of *novel* sentences is not introduced as a level of treatment until that time. Obviously, it is optimal if a patient is motivated to begin to use correct production of a limited number of sounds in conversations outside of the therapy session. If they are, they should certainly be encouraged to do so. However, their sentences will contain errors on non-target sounds and specific reinforcement for use of a specific sound should be provided. In other words, reinforcement would be "That was a good /p/ in chip," rather than "Good talking," especially if an error occurred on *ch*.

The clinician can assist very young children in generating sentences by guiding the child through descriptions of an object or picture, or by playing with two figures or dolls and starting a conversation between them. An excellent way of introducing sentences to children who can read is to use books, especially if the patient brings a favorite book to the session. Although they no longer have the clinician's auditory model, reading provides the visual cue of the printed letters. This type of visual cue, that is graphic, is useful for prompting the patient to include sounds already learned. Any word with an error should be repeated, and the sentence should be read again until it is read without errors. Appropriate reinforcement can be provided after each sentence and deferred for increasingly long intervals as success and confidence improve.

From Sentences to Conversation

Simple monologues can be used as a transitional step from sentences to conversation. In a monologue, the patient is given a topic and must speak about it for a specified amount of time, usually 30 seconds to a minute. By the time treatment reaches this level, production of all appropriate phonemes has reached a criterion of 90% accuracy at all previous levels. Therefore, the expectation is that the monologues will be spoken with accurate articulation. Monologue is introduced in order to elicit connected speech prior to dialogue (conversation) because it does not demand that the speaker formulate a response at the same time as they are monitoring speech production. It is, therefore, less linguistically and cognitively demanding. Monologues may be elicited using picture description or description of real or hypothetical situations.

When criterion is reached using monologue, the individual is ready to engage in dialogue. The clinician should be aware of the amount of cueing needed by the patient. When dialogue is first introduced, many patients need to be reminded to use their "good sounds" at intervals during the dialogue. Some need a reminder at the beginning of the conversation, others may need a cue upon entering the treatment room. Some individuals will respond to entering the speech room as a trigger for good speech, and will use their correct sounds upon entering. Obviously, this should be encouraged.

Carryover

The greatest hurdle faced by many patients is generalizing the speech production skills learned in treatment to their verbal interactions and conversations outside of the clinical situation. This is also the most challenging level of treatment because, by definition, the clinician is not present to provide cues or reinforcement. This level of the therapy process requires letting other people in the patient's world, who are still unaware, in on their secret—that they are capable of using correct speech. Contracts are a common therapy tool for increasing generalization to other situations. Other suggestions are described in Chapter 8.

A WORD ABOUT AUDITORY DISCRIMINATION

Some clinicians believe that auditory discrimination practice, also called ear training, is an essential first step in the therapy process. Proponents say that an individual cannot be expected to produce a sound if he or she cannot detect it. However, it is our experience that individuals are often unable to hear the difference between the target sound and their incorrect production until they have some experience in producing the sound correctly. This is consistent with theories of "categorial perception." Categorial perception explains a phenomenon of auditory perception that we hear sounds according to our own production. This explains exchanges such as this:

Clinician: Say 'sun.'
Child: Thun.
Clinician: Not 'thun,' 'sun.'
Child: That'th what I thaid. 'thun.'

When the patients have had experience in producing both their error and the correct target, most individuals are better able to hear the difference between them. Auditory discrimination is most important as a tool for the patient in later stages of treatment to monitor production of the target sound. Use of auditory discrimination as a procedure, rather than as a goal in and of itself, is discussed in Chapter 8.

TREATMENT OF ERRORS IN SPEAKERS
WITH PALATAL FISTULAE

It is desirable for treatment to be provided in the presence of a fully re-paired palate with no fistulae. However, this does not always occur. It is important to be sure that errors selected for treatment are not oblig-atory. A simple screening procedure is to have the patient say the sounds in question with the nares occluded. If the error disappears, it was obligatory. As stated previously, errors in this category are reduced intraoral pressure, nasal emission, and nasal turbulence. On the other hand, compensatory errors can always be corrected by speech therapy and compensatory adaptations usually can be corrected in spite of anatomic variations. Mid-dorsal palatal stops, which usually occur in the presence of large, central palatal fistulae, may be easier to correct if the fistula is occluded or repaired. The SLP should bring this situation to the attention of the cleft palate team so that the timing of repair can be considered. If repair will occur in a timely way, it may be worth-while to work on other errors until after repair, and then to correct the tongue-tip errors. On the other hand, if correction is not possible for 6 months or a year, treatment should proceed. The fistula can even be used as a placement target ("Put your tongue in front of the hole"). Liberal use of nasal occlusion to establish production can be used and faded out as described previously.

WHEN TO TREAT COMPENSATORY
ERRORS IN SPEAKERS WITH VPI

Most individuals with velopharyngeal insufficiency need physical cor-rection of VPI, either with a prosthetic appliance or pharyngoplasty. The goal of physical management is to provide velopharyngeal clo-sure. The speech goal of surgery is to eliminate hypernasality and the obligatory errors of nasal emission and reduced intraoral pressure. Correction of VPI does *not* change articulation in any other way. For years, clinicians and surgeons advocated performing pharyngoplasty prior to speech therapy to eliminate compensatory speech errors. They reasoned that VPI had to be corrected before therapy would be effec-tive because VPI was the predisposing factor in the development of the speech errors. Advances in diagnostic tools, specifically nasopha-ryngoscopy and multiview videofluoroscopy, permit observation of velopharyngeal motion during unimpeded connected speech and have led to an alternate view. It has been observed that glottal stops are usu-ally accompanied by little or no pharyngeal wall motion, and that nasal snorting is accompanied by outward velopharyngeal motion. The same speakers often exhibit normalized inward motion of the pharyngeal walls during correct oral consonant production, even when VPI is still present. Therefore, it is usually our recommendation that speech therapy to eliminate abnormal compensatory errors be accomplished before pharyngoplasty so that imaging of the VP region, necessary to plan appropriate surgery, can be done when the mechanism can be assumed to be functioning at its best (Golding-Kushner, 1989; Shprintzen, 1990).

It has been reported that surgical correction of VPI does not reduce the time of speech intervention necessary to completely eliminate compensatory articulation (Ysunza et al., 1996). Still, there are some individuals with VPI who seem to progress very slowly during articulation treatment and clinicians sometimes suspect that progress would be more rapid if the VPI was not present. These patients may benefit from the temporary use of a speech bulb appliance. This enables them to learn correct oral articulation without VPI and maintains the advantage of delaying surgery until velopharyngeal motion can be examined during correct speech. In many individuals, the speech bulb can be reduced gradually over a period of time with accompanying increase in velo-pharyngeal motion (McGrath & Anderson, 1990; Golding-Kushner et al., 1995). Speech bulb appliances may also be beneficial in patients who have to have surgery delayed for medical or other reasons, as well.

Some individuals have been told that speech has to be "relearned" following pharyngeal flap surgery or other pharyngoplasty. This is not the case. Individuals use the same pattern of articulation following surgery as they do before surgery. This means that if a speaker produces glottal stops before the operation, he or she will produce glottal stops after the operation, until taught otherwise. Similarly, if the speaker produces correct oral consonants before surgery, he or she will come out of surgery with good speech. In fact, they will sound better because the obligatory distortions and hypernasality should be gone. Glottal speakers tend to sound about the same postoperatively because nasal emission and reduced intraoral pressure are not significant factors in a glottal speech disorder, and hypernasality is not a major obstacle in terms of intelligibility.

HOW LONG SHOULD THERAPY TAKE?

Speech therapy to correct compensatory errors associated with cleft palate and VPI should be measured in months, not years. As stated earlier, it is usually possible to elicit correct production of isolated sounds during the stimulability testing that occurs during the evaluation. New speech behaviors at the word-imitation level should occur in one or two sessions. Moving from the word to phrase level should be possible within a month or two, if that long, and so on.

CHAPTER

8

Procedures and Materials

It should be obvious that procedures and materials are two separate things. Unfortunately, the difference is often blurred. Procedures are the steps that are followed to reach a specific goal. Materials are the things that are used to carry out a procedure. The term "reinforcement" refers to a procedure that is used after a response has occurred. The purpose of reinforcement is to increase the likelihood that a response will be repeated and learned. If significant progress has not occurred within 2 months, the clinician should consider changing the therapy schedule or the procedures being used.

REINFORCEMENT

As discussed in Chapter 3, behavior modification technique uses three types of contingency responses—positive reinforcement, negative reinforcement, and punishment. Positive reinforcement, a stimulus applied to a specific behavior, increases the likelihood that the behavior will increase in frequency. The opposite of positive reinforcement is punishment. Punishment is the application of an aversive stimulus that is intended to decrease the likelihood of the behavior being repeated. The effects of punishment are almost always transient and rarely extinguish undesirable behaviors. Negative reinforcement is the removal of an aversive stimulus that has the effect of increasing frequency of response. For example, if a child dislikes being in therapy, the therapy itself can be used as a negative reinforcer. The child may be told that the session can be shortened (i.e., removal of an aversive stimulus) if he or she gives the desired number of responses in a shorter period of time. This type of operant tends to be very effective because behaviors that are repeated more frequently in a shorter period of time tend to be learned faster. Another mechanism for eliminating undesirable behaviors is nonreinforcement. By ignoring behaviors, they will not be reinforced, and, therefore, are likely to be dropped.

In order to be most effective, reinforcement should be provided on a fixed interval schedule at first, then on a variable interval schedule as consistency of response improves. A fixed interval schedule is one that is predictable, such as a reward for every correct response (a 1:1 schedule), or a reward for every 5 correct responses (a 1:5 schedule). A 1:1 schedule should be used at first, then larger intervals such as 1:5. When the patient's response consistency is high, reinforcement should be provided on a variable or random schedule. Verbal reinforcement should always be provided, even when token reinforcement is used, and verbal reinforcement should be specific. Primary reinforcement (edibles) should be avoided if possible. It takes longer to chew a piece of cereal than to move a game piece, receive a sticker, or add a block to a tower. Secondary (token, game) reinforcement should be fun but very quick. Reinforcement must always be immediate to the response. Any delay may have the effect of reinforcing the wrong behavior (Table 8–1).

CLINICAL MATERIALS

Speech therapy for compensatory errors does not require elaborate or expensive materials. The clinician should have the following clinical items on hand: a table-top or wall-mounted mirror, large enough to see the therapist and child at same time (Figure 8–1), gloves, nose clips

---

TABLE 8–1 *Reinforcement*

1. Reinforcement schedule should be at fixed intervals at first, then at variable intervals as consistency of response improves.
2. Verbal reinforcement should be specific and immediate.
3. Primary reinforcement (edibles) should be avoided if possible. It takes longer to chew a piece of cereal or a raisin than to move a game piece or add a block to a tower.
4. Secondary reinforcement (tokens, games) should be fun but very quick.

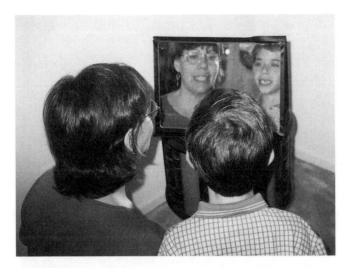

FIGURE 8–1. A mirror should be used that is large enough for the clinician and patient to see themselves and each other simultaneously.

(optional), nasal emission mirror or stethoscope, cotton balls, drinking straws, tape recorder, and audio cassettes. These items are used at all levels of treatment. All the types of cues used during stimulability testing (visual placement, visual airflow, manual, tactile, auditory, verbal) may also be used to elicit sounds and provide feedback during treatment. For example, the oral direction of airflow can be demonstrated and amplified using a drinking straw. The straw should be held with the top opening just below the maxillary central incisors. When the air is correctly centrally directed, a hissing sound will be emitted through the straw. Cotton balls can be used to demonstrate air pressure behind a /p/. A See-scape™ may be used with the nasal tip placed orally to provide visual feedback of oral air pressure during bilabial sound production (Figure 8–2).

At various times, nasal occlusion will be peformed by the clinician or patient. The clinician should use a gloved hand to hold the child's nose, or lightweight plastic nose clips can be used (Figure 8–3). The advantages of the nose clips are that they do not obstruct the view of the child's mouth. Young children may find them less threatening because they can help position them without being touched by the clinician, and can be left in place for several consecutive trials. Nose clips should be used only for a single patient to avoid contamination. They can be sent home for use during practice sessions.

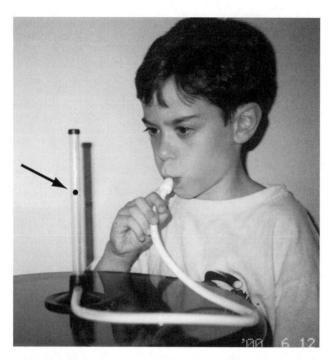

FIGURE 8–2. A See-scape™ can be used to provide visual feedback of oral airflow during production of labial plosives and fricatives. Here, production of /b/. Oral air pressure from the mouth at the plosive release causes the small piston in the verticle tube to rise.

THERAPY MATERIALS

Materials fall into two categories: materials used as part of the therapy process to elicit responses, and materials used for reinforcement tasks. Therapy is most efficient when the materials presented serve both functions. Different types of materials include cards, pictures, word lists, toys, board games, and computer games. In the following section, sample activities for using each will be described.

Pictures

There are many commercially available sets of picture cards designed to elicit specific target phonemes. These often have clear, easily recognizable pictures. They must be carefully sorted to allow selection of appropriate target words. Unfortunately, commercially available decks

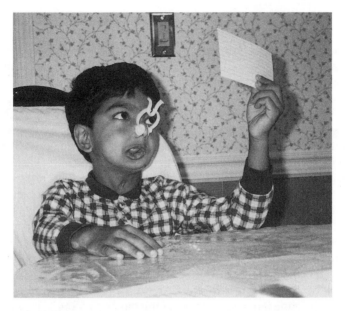

FIGURE 8–3. Nose clips provide sustained nasal occlusion during drills without interfering with speech or obstructing the clinician's view of the patient's mouth.

tend to target the most common error sounds such as /r, l, s, θ/ and have shared decks for less common errors such as /p, b/. Fewer companies have decks available for /t, d/, and it is very difficult to find picture sets for /h/ and /w/. Therefore, preparing materials to work on these sounds requires some creativity on the part of the clinician. Pictures can be found in picture dictionaries, children's books, and even supermarket circulars. Store circulars are often the best source of simple pictures for familiar target words such as "ham, pie, pea, tea," especially if a food theme is being used for a child working on both articulation and language goals. A picture of an owl from an animal book can be used to elicit "who." The clinician should have the target pictures ready before the session, so that valuable treatment time is not spent searching and cutting. Picture sets should be prepared for use by copying or cutting them and gluing them on blank index cards. The cards can be laminated to increase their durability. Copies of pictures should be given to the child for home practice. It is a poor use of home practice time and effort to have the child and parent search for particular pictures and cut them out. The clinician can locate appropriate target words much more quickly, and precious home practice time can be used for speech production, not busywork.

PLACEMENT OF MATERIALS

Regardless of the procedure used, placement of materials is an important consideration. Visual production cues obtained by watching the clinician's mouth are an important source of training. Therefore, it is important for the patient to watch the clinician's mouth during modeled production. Excess verbalization should be kept to a minimum, making it undesirable to constantly repeat "Look at me." A way to avoid this when using picture cues or small toys to be named is for the clinician to hold the stimulus object next to her mouth (Figure 8–4). The patient will turn their attention there to see the picture or toy, and requests for attention will not be necessary. If a physical object is not being used, the reinforcement object can be held beside the clinician's mouth while the word is said, or mouthed.

Holding the stimulus picture or object slightly above eye level of the patient is useful during the patient's production, especially when working on correction of mid-dorsal palatal stops (Figure 8–5). The patient will tip the head upward slightly to see the picture to be named, allowing the clinician a better view of the patient's mouth. This reduces the possibility of inadvertently reinforcing dorsal stops, which may be acoustically close to correctly produced tongue-tip sounds.

PROCEDURES

As stated above, procedures are the things the clinician does with the materials that are being used. When selecting procedures, the clinician must be certain that therapy time is used efficiently. The child is there because of a speech production problem. Teach them correct speech production.

Sample Activities Using Pictures

1. Matching Games

Children enjoy memory games in which sets of picture pairs are placed face down on a table and turned over two at a time. Another matching game is Go Fish, in which players ask each other for a specific picture. Depending on the level of treatment, the child can simply name the desired picture or use a carrier phrase to request it. These activities are appropriate beginning at a naming level, but are not appropriate when the patient is working on imitation of the clinician's model. In both matching activities, the cards provide the stimuli for the session and the game serves as a reinforcement activity. The clinician should count out the

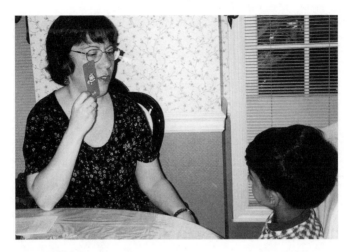

FIGURE 8–4. While working at an imitative level of therapy or when the patient still needs visual mouthing cues, the clinician holds stimulus materials next to her mouth so the patient will see the target word and benefit from visual cues for articulator placement at the same time.

number of picture pairs in use to determine how many repetitions are needed to achieve the goal of 100 for each session. Before the cards are put into play, the child should name each one using correct articulation a specified number of times. During play, the child should name or repeat each picture turned over a specified number of times, even if it is the clinician's "turn." If they ask why they have to say the words when it is not their turn, the answer is that the clinician does not need the speech practice and they do. This doubles the number of productions and optimizes the use of treatment time. The desired 100 correct productions in a session can be achieved as follows: if 20 pairs of pictures are used, naming each picture once before the game results in 40 productions. During the game, they name each picture turned over. If each picture is turned over 1 time, they reach 80. However, a match will not be made on each turn. The additional 20 will be elicited on the remaining trials. More speech practice can be elicited by having the child say each word twice in succession. This adds minimal time to the activity and will result in 200 correct productions per session. When cards are used with a patient at a phrase or sentence level of treatment, each response takes longer and more than 100 may be difficult to achieve. Phonetically appropriate carrier phrases should be introduced such as "I want _____," "Do you have _____?" or "I see a _____."

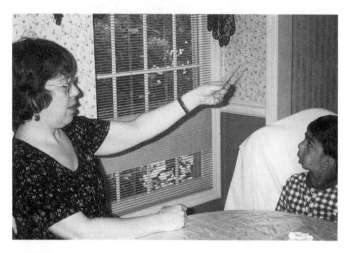

FIGURE 8–5. When the therapist's placement cues are no longer needed and the patient is working at a naming level of therapy, stimuli can be held slightly above eye level. This allows the clinician to see the patient's mouth more easily. This is especially useful for observing differences in tongue-tip position for alveolar, velar, and mid-dorsal palatal stops.

2. Playing Cards

School-aged children at the naming level or higher often enjoy card games played with traditional decks of cards, such as War, Rummy, Poker and Twenty-One. These games can easily be adapted for articulation therapy. The simplest way is with the use of articulation decks that, in addition to a picture for a target articulation sound, have a suit marking (heart, diamond, club, spade). The picture on every revealed card must be named with correct speech a designated number of times. If these cards are not available, regular cards can be used when the child is able to produce the sounds in all numbers (/w, t, θ, f, v, r, s, n, dʒ, kw, k, ŋ/) and suit shapes (/h, r, t, s, p, d, k, l/) or colors (/r, d, b, l, k/) correctly *and* is working at a level of treatment involving multiple target sounds. As with the matching card games, use of standard playing cards provides both the stimuli and reinforcement for the session.

3. Setting up a Homework Assignment

Setting up their homework book is a fun and useful task for children from about age 2^1/2 years. The therapist should have copies of the selected pictures in a pile and tell the child "These pictures are mine, but you can get all of them before you leave today." The child has to repeat or name each picture correctly five consecutive times. As the child names the picture, the therapist holds up a finger and says "Good." If an error is made before the fifth time, the count starts again. When the child names the picture correctly five consecutive times (the fingers on one hand), they are handed a glue stick to glue the picture into the speech homework book. If the child is distracted by the glue stick or is slow in applying glue to the picture, the clinician should apply the glue and give the picture to the child to stick on the designated page in the speech book, in a position of his or her choice. This activity continues until the desired number of pictures has been glued in the book. The pictures provide the stimulus material for the session, and the gluing or picture placement activity is the reinforcement task. It is quick and does not interfere with the flow of treatment. Ten pictures is a good number for most children to take for nightly home practice. This means that setting up the speech book for homework will be complete after a minimum of 50 correct productions, assuming all sequences of five were correct on the first trial. Depending on how much time is left in the session, the parent should be brought in and the child can show how he will produce "five correct in a row" at home. This will give the additional 50 target productions needed to reach 100. If services are provided at school, the child can review the task with the clinician ("Now show me how you will do this at home tonight"). If it can be arranged, the child should also show the classroom teacher what they are practicing. This is sometimes possible immediately after a session, but more often must be delayed until just before lunch or recess, or at some other time during the day that the child can have a few moments alone with the teacher to say each word correctly one or two times. In addition to providing additional speech practice for the child, it enables the classroom teacher to follow the child's progress at an earlier level of treatment than they are usually involved in, or even before they are generally aware of what is going on in speech therapy.

4. Picture Card Naming

At the early stages of treatment, cards can be used for imitation and naming practice. The clinician should hold the card near her mouth to be sure the child is watching for available visual cues and produce the word. The child should repeat the word. Specific verbal reinforcement should be provided. If needed, simple token reinforcement may also be introduced. Token reinforcement must be simple, immediate to the response, and quick to be efficient.

5. Minimal Pairs

Minimal pairs are words that differ in one phoneme, such as bye-tie, bye-bite, goat-coat, and pear-bear. When the child has enough phonemes in their repertoire to produce minimal pairs, use of paired pictures can provide an excellent vehicle to elicit specific sound production. Most speakers who produce glottal stops use them for all plosives. The use of minimal pairs creates the need to differentiate sounds because the contrasting phonemes convey meaning. This can be done in listening tasks and in production tasks, using auditory discrimination as a procedure to elicit correct consonant production.

TOYS

Young children respond well to the use of small toys, such as people and animal figures and familiar objects. Toys can be presented for play based on the sounds they can elicit. For example, when working on /h/ with a limited phonetic inventory, the toy set could consist of a home, hoe, hay, hill, hammer, hand, (doll clothes) hanger, owl that says "who," and a small Santa that says "ho ho." Other words introduced could be "here, hi, high."

When working at a syllable level, blocks or small balls can be used as they "talk" their way across the play area repeating target syllables such as "pa pa pa."

As children move up treatment levels and begin to use their new sounds in sentences and conversation, play with common objects is an excellent activity that encourages use of the new speech patterns in a natural way. For example, a miniature play house with a wide array of people, furniture, food items, and other props should be available. At first, the child can play while the clinician asks questions about the actions to elicit verbal responses. The clinician can also model play actions and encourage the child to try the actions, to describe them, and even to talk for the "characters." Like storytelling, this is an especially appropriate activity for children working on both articulation and language goals.

Using Toys for Token Reinforcement

Examples of token reinforcement are putting a marble in a cup, adding a single piece of track to a train set-up, and adding a block to a box or tower. A 1:1 reinforcement schedule should be used at first. However, it is most efficient to use a 1:5 reinforcement schedule: for every five correct responses, give one reinforcer. Some young children do not respond well to even that much delay and need a 1:1 schedule. When a 1:5 or greater schedule is possible, reinforcers might include coloring a segment of a picture or gluing a picture in the speech book for home practice. These activities are not recommended for the 1:1 schedule because they are more time consuming and reduce available speech time.

For children who can partially delay gratification, a mixed token-play system can be used. In this paradigm, pieces are collected on the 1:1 or 1:5 schedule for use in a game that is played at the end of the session, after the criterion of 100 correct productions is achieved. Examples are, collecting beans to play Don't Spill the Beans, placing plastic cubes in a frame to play Don't Break the Ice, and collecting logs to build a Lincoln Log structure. The strategy of setting aside pieces for subsequent play is also useful for children who are distracted by the reinforcement but want to play at the end of the session. The therapist can set aside a box, and place one of the pieces in the box on the appropriate reinforcement schedule. A play time is designated according to the child's age and ability to delay, such as after 10 pieces are in the box, after 10 minutes, or after 100 correct productions have been produced. At that time, the box can be given to the child for a short period of play, not to exceed 2 minutes. Then the pieces are removed from the child's view and speech productions resume.

BOOKS AND STORYTELLING

At the word level of treatment, books can be read to the child who, in turn, can be encouraged to finish sentences started by the clinician. The clinician can selectively omit words with the child's target sound(s). Also, pictures in the books can be used to elicit specific words or phrases. When the child is working at a sentence or conversational level, picture sequences can be used to elicit speech. For young children, the sequences should be familiar and might include families engaged in everyday activities such as cooking, doing laundry or playing hide-and-seek. If they do not elaborate, the clinician can ask questions to elicit more complex information, that is, responses containing the target sounds and details. Then, the clinician can tell a story about the pictures, using as many target words as possible. Following this modeling, the child can be asked to retell the story, which should result in a more elaborate response than their spontaneous story. Parents should receive some training in procedures for storytelling tasks from picture cards and books. Once trained, these are excellent home activities for language as well as articulation in sentences, monologue and dialogue.

Older children who are able to read also enjoy storytelling activities. They can begin by reading a story, which allows them to benefit from graphic cues for their target sound, then answering specific questions about the story to elicit target words. They can then retell the story to produce a monologue using correctly articulated sounds. These are also examples of activities that can be used to integrate articulation and language goals when appropriate.

WORD LISTS

Word lists are useful for older children and save time when picture sets for a specific target sound are not available. Lists can also include words not easily depicted, and phonetically appropriate words that the child may have on spelling lists or in other subject areas at school. Integrating vocabulary and content words from other aspects of the child's life is critical for facilitating carryover, and also helps make the speech therapy process more anchored in the real world of the child and family. Words can be printed on index cards for use in card games described above, or written in a book for quick production tasks. Using printed words adds a graphic cue to the other types of speech production cues provided.

GAMES

Children love to play board games, and they can be integrated into speech sessions easily. However, the clinician must be careful to ensure that the game is the reinforcer, not the main focus. Speech production opportunities must be maximized. For example, at the word level, each turn should consist of five correct productions of a target word followed by a move on the board. If the game includes a spinner or dice, the child can be required to say the number of words rolled five times each to maximize speech production. The pawn is moved after the words are said correctly. If the child rolled a six, he will have said 30 words correctly (six words, five times each) to take one turn.

Some games require a lot of talking and lend themselves well to doubling as both the speech stimulus and reinforcement activity. This is appropriate when the child has a sufficient repertoire of correctly produced phonemes. A popular game for this purpose is Guess Who? which is also a frequently used language therapy tool. In this game, each of two players has a tray with pictures of people. Each player draws a card depicting one of the people and the players must ask each other yes/no questions to collect clues to guess the identity of the other player's "mystery" person. The patient should be required to use specific carrier phrases to ask and answer questions. For example, the carrier phrase used to ask questions by a child working on /s/ and /r/ might be "Does your mystery person have . . . . . ?" The required answer would be "Yes, my mystery person has . . . . . ," or "No, my mystery person does not have . . . . ."

Another popular game that requires talking is Battleship. It is similar to Guess Who in that the players must guess what is on the other player's hidden board. The ability to correctly produce letter names and numbers is required to use this game effectively.

The procedures described are easily adapted to other games, and children are often very enthusiastic about coming to therapy with a new game or toy from home. The designated carrier phrases can be put into their speech homework book, and homework at this level of treatment might consist of playing the game every day with a parent using the required phrases. Very few children complain about this type of speech homework!

Most of the preceding examples described games for two people. While individual treatment is optimal, many children are in group therapy settings. If there are two children, they play against each other. If more children are present, games can be adapted for use by forming teams. Child A would be the spokesperson for the team on one turn, and child B would be the spokesperson for the team on the next turn. They could consult with each other to decide what to guess. The obvious disadvantage of this is that each child has fewer speech opportunities. That, of course, is a major disadvantage of all group therapy arrangements.

AUDITORY DISCRIMINATION AS A PROCEDURE

There is one exception to the statement that the patient should name each picture, even on the clinician's turn. Auditory discrimination tasks are helpful at the phrase and sentence levels of treatment to facilitate the development of self-monitoring skills that are important in establishing carryover. By the time he or she has reached this level of treatment, the child has established the ability to produce the sound correctly and should be able to hear the difference between the error and target. The child can be assigned the role of therapist on the clinician's turn. The clinician should name the picture or say the target phrase using correct articulation on some turns and produce the patient's error on some turns. The patient must act as therapist, tell the clinician if the word or phrase was produced correctly or not, and if not, correct the error.

HOME PRACTICE

For very young children, parents should be trained in techniques to integrate language and speech stimulation into daily activities. Older children who are learning articulation skills, especially those who are working to eliminate a compensatory speech disorder, must have an opportunity to review and rehearse skills taught in therapy. The most effective way to accomplish this is through the use of structured home practice sessions. When patients and parents complain about "speech homework," I offer a deal: if the child does not speak *at all* for the entire day, they do not have to practice correct speech. However, most children talk a great deal between 7 a.m. when they wake up and 8 p.m. or later, when they go to sleep. This means they are "rehearsing" their speech errors over and over for 13 or more hours. It is not unreasonable to set aside 3 to 5 minutes to practice correct speech.

Homework assignments should be structured so that maximum correct practice can occur in a short time. Speech production tasks *must* always be done by the child in the presence of an adult who can listen, discriminate the correct and incorrect productions, and cue the child effectively to correct any errors on target sounds. Speech homework cannot be done with a 10-year-old sibling, who may have good intention but lacks the skill to implement the tasks as necessary. If the adult helper cannot do these tasks, there is a risk of reinforcing incorrect productions for several days at a time.

In order to optimize success, homework assignments should trail therapy tasks by two sessions. For example, let's say the child produced /s/ in isolation and in CV syllables at Session 1. Homework for this session is to purchase a speech notebook, if not provided by the clinician. He produced CV syllables and CVC words at Session 2. There is no homework after this session. At Session 3, the child continues with CVC words. There are two homework assignments after this session. Both assignments are to be done daily. The first assignment is to produce /s/ correctly in isolation five consecutive correct times per day with the nose closed, followed by five consecutive /s/ sounds with the nose opened. The second assignment is to repeat ten CV syllables that are written in the book after his helper, five consecutive correct times. Homework is based on the tasks that were completed successfully two sessions earlier. The five isolated /s/ productions and 50 syllables will take about 2 minutes per day to perform if the child has few errors. If there are more errors, the practice session will take longer because the assignment is five *consecutive* correct productions. If the child makes an error, the count for that syllable begins again. At most, homework will take 5 minutes. The homework task is done with the child prior to the end of the session at which it is assigned, and timed. The child is shown that he can complete the task in this very short period of time. This reduces excuses for not doing homework, such as being too busy, having other homework, and so on.

Parents who accompany the child to speech therapy can receive training in how to help the child with speech homework effectively and training to discriminate between the desired target sound and the child's compensatory errors. Sometimes, parents need additional support in this process. There is also a need to convey this information and training to caregivers who are not in direct contact with the clinician. It may be useful for the clinician to videotape the part of the speech therapy session in which she explains to the child what to do for homework. The SLP and child should then do an entire 3–5 homework assignment. The child and parent can watch the 5 minute tape together that evening before practicing, so that both are sure of the assignment. The parent can see and hear the therapist's responses to the child's correct and incorrect speech attempts, and the clinician can model elicitation and reinforcement procedures. Harding-Bell (2000) suggested videotaping entire speech-language therapy sessions for the child and parent to watch at home. Children love to watch themselves on T.V., and, if they are encouraged to respond to the therapist with themselves on T.V., it is almost like having an extra treatment session.

The homework book should contain helper "sign lines." There is one line for each day until the next session, including the day of the current session. After each practice, the helper, not the child, should sign to indicate completion. If a day is missed, the line should be left blank so that the clinician knows how many practice sessions occurred. If the child does an extra practice to make up for a missed day, the correct date should be marked in. It is important to explain to the child and parent that the purpose of the signatures is not to "check up" on the child. It is to provide the clinician with accurate practice information to help understand progress or lack of progress. Each session begins by doing the homework that was completed for that day. If the child makes errors on many trials and the book has not been signed, the poor performance can be understood. If the book has all the lines signed, there are several possibilities. The child may have been practicing errors, the assignment may have been too difficult, or the family may have cheated and signed without practicing. The child and helper must understand that truthful information is crucial in planning therapy tasks and subsequent homework. In this example, the clinician must determine if the helper needs additional training to reinforce correct sounds, if the assignment needs to trail by three sessions instead of two, or if the family needs to understand the importance of practice and "truth in reporting."

Here is another example of how the "sign-lines" provide important information. Let's say the child usually practices three of four days and does well. The one day off did not seem to make a difference. He then practices only two of four days and accuracy during the next session is poor. The clinician, child, and helper have evidence that the extra day of practice makes a difference and the child must practice at least three of every four days. This helps maintain compliance for homework.

Another important homework tip is that the most important day to do homework is the day of the session. Some people think it is odd to say that 2 minutes of home practice is important if the child just spent 30 minutes with the clinician. However, after that session is the time at which correct production is fresh in the child's mind and the assignment is clear. Therefore, the night of the therapy session is a critical practice night.

Written instructions given with the first homework assignment should also include a reminder to add "sign lines" and continue the same homework if a session is missed for any reason. This increases the possibility that the child and parent will continue to practice even if—especially if—a session is missed. It is always amazing that seemingly intelligent children and parents verbalize their understanding of the importance of daily practice yet, after a missed session, will say they did not continue to practice because there was no assignment!

Homework must be continued during school vacations. Also, it should be clear to children receiving treatment at school that declarations of "homework free nights" do not apply to speech homework. Continuity and repetition are essential.

Homework assignments should be clear and specific. In order to maximize speech production and minimize the time to complete the assignment, a drill approach is appropriate. When criterion is reached and production is accurate, it takes 2 minutes to repeat 10 words five times each. Keeping in mind that homework is based on tasks that are close to criterion because they trail therapy, the child can produce 50 correct words in 2 minutes. On the other hand, cutting pictures from a magazine with certain initial consonant sounds or doing a hidden pictures task may prolong the homework time to 30 minutes or even more, and with minimal talking needed during that time. That is a lot of work for very little speech return and not worth the effort. A sample homework assignment and signature page is shown in Figure 8–6.

The clinician should provide training to parents to enable them to assist in a helpful way with homework assignments. The training should include instruction on how to provide appropriate, specific positive reinforcement for correct productions, as well as encouragement when effort is shown but the sound is incorrect. Ear training for the parent may be necessary to be certain that the parent can hear the difference between the target sound and error sound. The procedures that were described for training parents of infants in home programs are also effective for parents of older children, and the reader may refer back to Chapter 3 for more information.

CARRYOVER

Some young children make the jump from good speech during therapy to good speech in other situations on their own. Something just

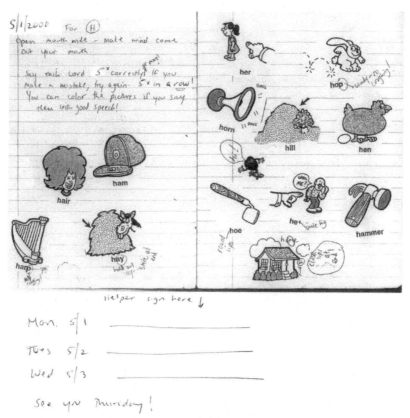

FIGURE 8–6. Page from a patient's speech homework book. Included are sound production instructions for the parents to use if cueing is needed, a specific practice assignment, target words for the patient to practice, and signature lines ("sign lines") for the child's adult helper to sign after each practice session. Most of these illustrations are taken from *Webbers Jumbo Articulation Drill Book* by & M. Thomas Webber & Sharon Webber, 1993 Greenville, SC: Super Duper School Company. Copyright 1993 by Bristol, Hart, and S. Savage. Reprinted with permission.

seems to "click" and they take off with correct articulation. Most children, however, need a guided journey into the world of good speech outside of therapy.

Daily home practice with a parent or other consistent speech helper sets up a logical beginning point for carryover tasks. For example, homework might consist of reading a page of a favorite book out loud to their helper using correct articulation, then telling about it with good articulation. Children who have school homework can be instructed to read out loud from a paper or book assigned by the classroom teacher for the desired duration. They are often both surprised and intrigued by the suggestion to do speech homework at the same time as their reading, math, or science work. What a novel idea! Using good speech during another task. This is an excellent starting point for encouraging carryover of correct speech to nonclinical settings. It also eliminates another popular excuse for not doing speech homework ("I forgot my speech book.") The author worked with a child in a public school who came to the speech room and had inadvertently brought her math notebook instead of her speech book. Eager to miss speech and return to her classroom, she offered to go retrieve the correct book, which was in a room on the other side of the building. She was surprised when she was told the book she had brought would suffice, and to start reading. She protested that it was a math book. She was told to read. Her articulation immediately returned to its pre-therapy, error-filled pattern. She was stopped and told to use her good speech. She proceeded to read each of the math problems and answers with correct articulation. It was the first time it had occurred to her that there was a connection between the work going on in the speech room and the rest of her world.

Contracts are a common therapy tool for increasing generalization to other situations. The patient and clinician write down specific speech criteria to be met in specific situations out of the therapy situation. These usually begin at home with the speech helper, but must also be developed to bring the patient's correct speech into the classroom and other speaking situations. Examples are using correct articulation for 5 minutes before bedtime when talking with a parent, or using correct /s/ sounds in the entire sentence when answering a question during a math lesson. If the child is old enough, they can keep track of which contracts were met and which fell short. Otherwise, a parent or teacher may have to be enlisted to provide reinforcement and to help the child keep track.

Children in school-based therapy have many carryover opportunities throughout the day that can be monitored indirectly by the clinician. A letter can be sent to all the child's teachers (classroom, specialty, etc.) explaining that the child is now able to say the ____ sound(s) and is learning to use it correctly when the clinician is not present. They can be asked to agree on some subtle cue that they can give the child as a reminder or as a reinforcer. The signal should be something that will be understood by the child but not be obvious to other students, to avoid making the child feel self-conscious about the process. For example, the teacher might call on the child, then scratch their ear as a signal to the child to read with good sounds.

The amount of time the child is expected to use good speech out of the therapy room is gradually increased. The parent should understand that the contracted period, whether 5 minutes or 3 hours, represents the time during which they can remind the child about using correct speech. Reminders outside of that time frame might be interpreted as "nagging" by the child and resisted. Eventually, the correct speech becomes second nature and automatic.

The SLP's responsibility does not end at the end of the speech session. If the child is not generalizing correct articulation, even when the process is broken down into short intervals, the patient, parents, and teachers should be brought into the session to formulate and formalize a plan. Additional suggestions for troubleshooting some common therapy problems are listed in Table 8–2.

TABLE 8–2 *Suggestions for Troubleshooting Common Problems*

Problem	Possible Solution
Producing glottal stops	• increase frequency of therapy • increase drill format to elicit more responses
Can't get rid of tongue backing	• check for palatal fistula • introduce /θ/
Can't get carryover without glottals	• break goals down into smaller steps • increase frequency of therapy
Velopharyngeal closure good on nasopharyngoscopy during limited speech sample, but there is no carryover and speech is hypernasal	• do careful speech analysis of nasopharynoscopy
Nasopharyngoscopy shows closure on single words or 2–3 words but longer speech strings show pulsing open/close	• r/o VCFS, • may still need pharyngoplasty
Producing sounds on inhalation instead of exhalation	• use t to facilitate s, • practice inhalation without sound followed by sound on exhalation
Producing lip smacking for bilabials	• teach airflow management, not only lip placement • check velopharyngeal closure

CHAPTER

9

Evaluation and Therapy Techniques to Avoid

When treating a child with compensatory articulation errors, it is as important to know what techniques to avoid as it is to know useful procedures. This knowledge can save time and effort, and helps ensure that treatment is not only effective, but also efficient. Many techniques have been applied by clinicians to the speech problems associated with velopharyngeal insufficiency but they have not been applicable for two basic reasons. First, many of these procedures were developed long ago when our understanding of the physiology of speech was limited. Procedures such as blowing or palatal massage were first recommended before scientists and clinicians had the modern instrumentation that has allowed us to observe velopharyngeal valving disorders in a systematic manner. Other techniques, such as the use of sign language or oral-motor therapy, have been borrowed from their application with other pathologies on a purely theoretical basis. There have been no rigorous scientific investigations that would suggest their advantage. Stated more strongly, these techniques have a long history of failure. On the other hand, the direct articulation therapy techniques described throughout this volume have been applied successfully to thousands of patients with a high degree of success.

ORAL-MOTOR EXERCISES

Exercises intended to increase lip, tongue, or jaw strength are inappropriate for several reasons. Strength of the articulators is not the reason for the errors.[1] The lack of lip and tongue use during speech may give a false impression of weakness. It is characteristic of speakers producing glottal stops to omit lip and tongue movement because, having valved the air at the level of the glottis, these movements have no purpose. In other words, omission of lip and tongue movement is caused by an error in learning and not to weakness of the muscles. Even most patients with very severe glottal stop speech disorders have normal tongue tip activity during production of nasal /n/ and normal bilabial closure for nasal /m/. It should be obvious that if tongue movement/ elevation is sufficient for /n/, it is sufficient for the oral cognates /t, d, s, l/ (Golding-Kushner, 1995). Therapists often do exercises to increase the range of motion of lip movement so that the speaker can move the tongue between the angles of the mouth, around the circumference of the mouth, protrude, and even elevate it beyond the lips to the nose. However, there are no speech sounds that require these movements, raising a question about the purpose of teaching these movements as part of a speech therapy program. Furthermore, there is not a proven relationship between strength of individual oral structures and accuracy of articulation.

New programs and therapeutic techniques designed to improve speech in specific populations are frequently described in journals and at professional conferences. It is important to analyze the rationale and goals of these programs, and to consider whether or not the techniques advocated are consistent with the needs of children with abnormal compensatory articulation errors. In most cases, they are not.

PALATAL AND VELOPHARYNGEAL EXERCISES

Another category of exercises to be avoided are those intended to increase palatal motion and velopharyngeal closure. These include palatal strengthening exercises, icing, palatal massage, nasal lavage, stroking, and even electrical stimulation. There is absolutely no relationship between the frequency and complexity of movements in the vocal tract during speech and nonspeech activities (Duffy, 1995; Johns, 1985; Robin et al., 1997). In fact, EMG activity of the velopharyngeal

---

[1]Strength of the articulators should not be confused with strength of articulatory contacts.

muscles is entirely different during speech and nonspeech activities (Trigos et al., 1988; Ysunza et al., 1999). Not surprisingly, there is no evidence that these activities result in improved velopharyngeal closure during speech or in decreased hypernasality (Powers & Starr, 1974; Ruscello, 1982; Starr, 1990; Van Demark & Hardin, 1990).

BLOWING EXERCISES

Blowing exercises, sucking, swallowing, gagging, and cheek puffing have also been suggested as useful in improving or strengthening velopharyngeal closure and speech. However, multiview videofluoroscopy has shown that velopharyngeal movements for these nonspeech functions differ from velopharyngeal movement for speech in the same speaker (Shprintzen et al., 1975). Improving velopharyngeal motion for these tasks does not result in improved resonance or speech. These procedures simply do not work and the premises and rationales behind them are scientifically unsound.

The purpose of soft palate movement and velopharyngeal closure appears to be to provide oral pressure for the production of pressure consonants. Further, electromyographic (EMG) activity to levator palatini increases as oral pressure increases (Kuehn & Moon, 1994). Thus, the best "palatal exercise" is speech.

APRAXIA PROGRAMS AND PROTOCOLS

Because of their lack of use of the lips and tongue, clinicians often attempt to apply procedures designed to improve organization of motor speech control in speakers with apraxia. It is important to understand that the lack of articulator movement in this population is not caused by apraxia. "Apraxia" is defined in Singular's Illustrated Dictionary of Speech-Language Pathology as the "inability to voluntarily execute a learned sequence of motor actions." They define "apraxia of speech" as a "neuromotor articulatory speech disorder caused by brain damage resulting in faulty planning, programming, or sequencing of the sounds of speech." Finally, they define "verbal apraxia" as a "primary deficit in planning the speech act, resulting in inconsistent phonemic distortions and substitutions with oral groping behaviors for voluntary verbal motor acts, but without muscular weakness or paralysis." (Singh & Kent, 2000, p. 15) *None* of these descriptions applies to individuals with compensatory articulation errors. Unfortunately, children with cleft palate speech, especially those with VCFS are often misdiagnosed as apraxic. As stated earlier, lack of movement of the lips and tongue during production of compensatory speech substitutions is caused by an error in learning and a change in the place of articulation. It is *not* caused by any of the parameters associated with apraxia. Therefore, treatment protocols designed to reduce the effects of apraxia should not be expected to be effective. If certain techniques that are part of these protocols seem to be appropriate for a particular child, it is reasonable to borrow from a program and use a technique or two. However, the clinician must be cautious in this regard.

SIGN LANGUAGE

The use of sign language has been advocated by some SLPs "to reduce frustration" and "to improve communication" for children with cleft palate speech and for children with delayed speech, including those diagnosed with velo-cardio-facial syndrome (Scherer & D'Antonio, 1998). Glottal stop speech disorders are errors in speech learning and speech production. Reducing frustration has merits, but it does not improve speech production, nor does it make the child more receptive to speech therapy. Glottal stops do not represent a limitation of speech production ability in the way that apraxia does. Furthermore, if the adults pay close attention they can see that a compensatory speech disorder is not an expressive language disorder, but rather a speech production problem. Therefore, teaching sign language does not address the problem. It seems highly inefficient to spend time teaching signs when that same time could be spent improving the speech production skills (Golding-Kushner & Shprintzen, 1998). Signing diverts attention and focus from the speech production problem and solution. It is like teaching the child a foreign language. Some advocates say that sign and speech can be taught simultaneously. However, with the emphasis on using nasal occlusion as a therapy technique, the SLP's hands should not be occupied with making signs. In addition, teaching sign requires the child to attend to the clinician's hands and their own hands, rather than the clinician's mouth and use of their own tongue and lips. Also, in most instances, children are able to communicate their needs by pointing and natural gesturing, which is encouraged because all children (and adults) gesture. Schools may not have the patience for this, and may advocate for the use of sign language to improve communication with the teacher. However, they are missing the boat and advocating an abnormal compensatory strategy added to another, rather than getting to the root of the problem—the speech production. Changes in speech ultimately result from direct therapy and increases in treatment schedule, not in the addition of signing to the list of goals.

PHONOLOGICAL ANALYSIS

Compensatory speech errors are mistakes in speech production, not in the organization of speech at a linguistic level. Elaborate and time consuming phonological analyses of the speech pattern do not contribute to understanding the articulation disorder. However, as noted earlier, the clinician should look at patterns of errors, not just individual sound substitutions when planning treatment. By definition, glottal stops and mid-dorsal palatal stops are "backing" errors. Phonological analysis adds nothing to this knowledge and is, therefore, a waste of time. Traditional analysis of errors that considers place, manner, and voicing of error and correctly produced sounds provides specific information that is useful in planning treatment. Groups of sounds with common features (such as bilabial plosives or the larger group of anterior plosives that included bilabial and lingua-alveolar stops) may be targeted together in therapy.

In addition, compensatory disorders often include glottal stops and other maladaptive errors that were described in Chapter 3. Phonological analysis does not have a "rule" that incorporates those other errors. "Glottal stop replacement" does not account for nasal snorting and pharyngeal stops, pharyngeal fricatives, or even for obligatory errors. Thus, the system is inadequate for classifying this type of speech disorder.

A FINAL WORD

The purpose of articulation therapy is to improve articulation. Procedures borrowed from other disciplines, or from treatment regimes that are effective for other communication disorders, should not be expected to have the same excellent results as can be achieved using direct articulation therapy. It is important for the clinician to remain focused on the goal of treatment and implement the most effective and efficient procedures to achieve that goal. The most effective and efficient way to use therapy time is to correct articulation errors and establish strong articulatory contacts. It is a poor and inefficient use of time to teach alternative communication strategies or to spend time on general intelligibility issues, such as rate reduction. The therapy goal is not just intelligible speech. The goal is *correct* speech. When articulation is correct, speech will be fully intelligible. Parents and clinicians who have spent months or even years using oral-motor therapy techniques, blowing exercises, or the other ill-advised procedures described, tend to be defensive about the progress in speech they eventually hear. They don't recognize that the sound that finally emerged after protracted treatment could have, in most cases, been elicited more quickly and simply.

Perhaps the most convincing testimony regarding procedures that work and do no not work comes from parents who have been through the proverbial mill with their children. On more than one occasion, parents have stated that their child demonstrated no speech improvement with a clinician intent on oral-motor exercises and sign language. When they switched therapists to one doing direct articulation therapy, there was dramatic improvement in 6 months. One of them wrote, "Yes, she's still hypernasal, but the improvement is phenomenal. I'm beginning to wonder if she'll even need surgery. Her newest word is 'purple' and even strangers can understand it." The parent of a child with VCFS wrote, "I can only tell you what worked for us. When we increased the drill format of speech therapy to four times per week we began to see great improvement. I also did a lot of work at home, just a few minutes at a time, but stuck to the drill . . . . We had the issue of being able to articulate during therapy and slipping back into the bad habits in conversation. Time seemed to fix that. Lots of practice worked for us. Within a year, all the errors were corrected. We now do only language therapy."

CHAPTER

10

Communication Disorders in Velo-Cardio-Facial Syndrome and Other Special Groups

VELO-CARDIO-FACIAL SYNDROME

Velo-cardio-facial syndrome (VCFS) (Figure 10–1) is one of the most common syndromes associated with cleft palate (Shprintzen, 2000). VCFS is a genetic condition caused by a small deletion on chromosome 22 and is also referred to as 22q11.2 deletion syndrome. VCFS has also been called DiGeorge sequence. There are over 180 features associated with VCFS (Table 10–1) and severe speech and language problems and learning disabilities are among the most common (Shprintzen et al., 1978; Golding-Kushner et al., 1985; Golding-Kushner, 1991; Kok and Solman, 1995; Scherer et al., 1999; D'Antonio et al., 2000; Shprintzen, 2000). Furthermore, the developmental pattern of the speech, language and learning patterns in children with VCFS may be unique and may require specialized intervention strategies (Scherer et al., 1999; Shprintzen, 2000; D'Antonio et al., 2000). Therefore, knowledge of the patterns of communication impairment in children with VCFS and effective, efficient intervention procedures is of great importance to SLPs.

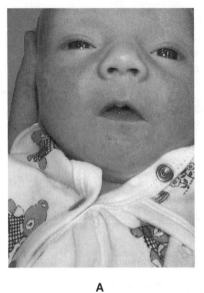

A

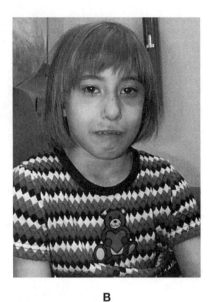

B

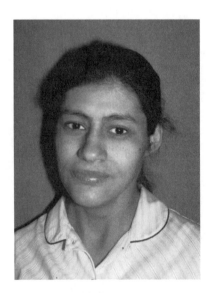

C

FIGURE 10-1. Facial appearance that is characteristic of velo-cardio-facial syndrome in a baby (**A**), child (**B**) and adult (**C**).

TABLE 10-1. *Velo-cardio-facial Syndrome: Specialist Fact Sheet (2000)*

Velo-cardio-facial syndrome (VCFS), also known as **Shprintzen syndrome,** sometimes presenting as the **DiGeorge sequence,** is caused by a deletion of a small segment of the long arm of chromosome 22. It is one of the most common genetic disorders in humans. The following list shows the anomalies which have been found in VCFS. No findings have a 100% frequency, but all occur with sufficient frequency to warrant assessment if suspected. For more information go to this URL: *http://www.vcfsef.org/facts.html*

Craniofacial/Oral Findings
1. Overt, submucous or occult submucous cleft palate
2. Retrognathia (retruded lower jaw)
3. Platybasia (flat skull base)
4. Asymmetric crying facies in infancy
5. Structurally asymmetric face
6. Functionally asymmetric face
7. Vertical maxillary excess (long face)
8. Straight facial profile
9. Congenitally missing teeth
10. Small teeth
11. Enamel hypoplasia (primary dentition)
12. Hypotonic, flaccid facies
13. Downturned oral commissures
14. Cleft lip (uncommon)
15. Microcephaly
16. Small posterior cranial fossa

Eye Findings
17. Tortuous retinal vessels
18. Suborbital congestion ("allergic shiners")
19. Strabismus
20. Narrow palpebral fissures
21. Posterior embryotoxin
22. Small optic disk
23. Prominent corneal nerves
24. Cataract
25. Iris nodules
26. Iris coloboma (uncommon)
27. Retinal coloboma (uncommon)
28. Small eyes
29. Mild orbital hypertelorism
30. Mild orbital dystopia
31. Puffy eyelids

TABLE 10-1. *Continued*

Ear/Hearing Findings
32. Overfolded helix
33. Attached lobules
34. Protuberant, cup-shaped ears
35. Small ears
36. Mildly asymmetric ears
37. Frequent otitis media
38. Mild conductive hearing loss
39. Sensori-neural hearing loss
40. Ear tags or pits (uncommon)
41. Narrow external ear canals

Nasal Findings
42. Prominent nasal bridge
43. Bulbous nasal tip
44. Mildly separated nasal domes (appearing bifid)
45. Pinched alar base, narrow nostrils
46. Narrow nasal passages

Cardiac Findings
47. VSD (Ventricular septal defect)
48. ASD (Atrial septal defect)
49. Pulmonic atresia or stenosis
50. Tetralogy of Fallot
51. Right sided aorta
52. Truncus arteriorsus
53. PDA (patent ductus arteriosus)
54. Interrupted aorta
55. Coarctation of the aorta
56. Aortic valve anomalies
57. Aberrant subclavian arteries
58. Vascular ring
59. Anomalous origin of carotid artery
60. Transposition of the great vessels
61. Tricuspid atresia

Vascular Anomalies
62. Medially displaced internal carotid arteries
63. Tortuous, kinked, absent, or accessory internal carotids
64. Jugular vein anomalies
65. Absence of vertebral artery (unilateral)
66. Low bifurcation of common carotid
67. Tortuous or kinked vertebral arteries
68. Reynaud's phenomenon
69. Small veins
70. Circle of Willis anomalies

TABLE 10-1. *Continued*

Neurologic and Brain Findings
71. Periventricular cysts (mostly at anterior horns)
72. Small cerebellar vermis
73. Cerebellar hypoplasia/dysgenesis
74. White matter UBOs (unidentified bright objects)
75. Generalized hypotonia
76. Cerebellar ataxia
77. Seizures
78. Strokes
79. Spina bifida/meningomyelocele
80. Mild developmental delay
81. Enlarged Sylvian fissure

Pharyngeal/Laryngeal/Airway Findings
82. Upper airway obstruction in infancy
83. Absent or small adenoids
84. Laryngeal web (anterior)
85. Large pharyngeal airway
86. Laryngomalacia
87. Arytenoid hyperplasia
88. Pharyngeal hypotonia
89. Asymmetric pharyngeal movement
90. Thin pharyngeal muscle
91. Unilateral vocal cord paresis

Abdominal/Kidney/Gut
92. Hypoplastic/aplastic kidney
93. Cystic kidneys
94. Inguinal hernias
95. Umbilical hernias
96. Malrotation of bowel (single case)
97. Hepatoblastoma (single case)
98. Diaphragmatic hernia (single case)
99. Anal anomalies (displaced, imperforate)

Limb Findings
100. Small hands and feet
101. Tapered digits
102. Short nails
103. Rough, red, scaly skin on hands and feet
104. Morphea
105. Contractures
106. Triphalangeal thumbs
107. Polydactyly (both preaxial and postaxial)
108. Soft tissue syndactyly

TABLE 10-1. *Continued*

Problems in Infancy
109. Feeding difficulty, failure-to-thrive
110. Nasal vomiting
111. Gastroesophageal reflux
112. Nasal regurgitation
113. Irritability
114. Chronic constipation (not Hirschsprung megacolon)

Speech/Language
115. Severe hypernasality
116. Severe articulation impairment
117. Language impairment (usually mild delay)
118. Velopharyngeal insufficiency (usually severe)
119. Dyspraxia
120. High pitched voice
121. Hoarseness

Cognitive/Learning
122. Learning disabilities (math concept, reading comprehension)
123. Concrete thinking, difficulty with abstraction
124. Drop in IQ scores in school years (test artifact)
125. Borderline normal intellect
126. Occasional mild mental retardation
127. Attention deficit hyperactivity disorder

Miscellaneous Anomalies
128. Spontaneous oxygen desaturation without apnea
129. Thrombocytopenia
130. Bernard-Soulier disease
131. Juvenile rheumatoid arthritis

Psychiatric/Psychological
132. Bipolar affective disorder
133. Manic depressive illness and psychosis
134. Rapid or ultrarapid cycling of mood disorder
135. Mood disorder
136. Depression
137. Hypomania
138. Schizoaffective disorder
139. Impulsiveness
140. Flat affect
141. Dysthymia
142. Cyclothymia
143. Social immaturity
144. Obsessive compulsive disorder

TABLE 10-1. *Continued*

145. Generalized anxiety disorder
146. Phobias

Immunologic
147. Frequent upper respiratory infections
148. Frequent lower airway disease (pneumonia, bronchitis)
149. Reduced T cell populations
150. Reduced thymic hormone
151. Reactive airway disease

Genitourinary
152. Hypospadias
153. Cryptorchidism
154. G-U reflux

Endocrine
155. Hypocalcemia
156. Hypoparathyroidism
157. Pseudohypoparathyroidism
158. Hypothyroidism
159. Mild growth deficiency, relative small stature
160. Absent, hypoplastic thymus
161. Hypoplastic pituitary gland

Skeletal/Muscle/Orthopedic/Spine
162. Scoliosis
163. Hemivertebrae
164. Spina bifida occulta
165. Butterfly vertebrae
166. Fused vertebrae (mostly cervical)
167. Tethered spinal cord
168. Syrinx
169. Osteopenia
170. Sprengel's anomaly, scapular deformation
171. Talipes equinovarus
172. Small skeletal muscles
173. Joint dislocations
174. Chronic leg pains
175. Flat foot arches
176. Hyperextensible/lax joints
177. Extra ribs
178. Rib fusion

TABLE 10-1. *Continued*

Skin/Integument
179. Abundant scalp hair
180. Thin appearing skin (venous patterns easily visible)

Secondary Sequences/Associations
181. Robin sequence
182. DiGeorge sequence
183. Potter sequence
184. CHARGE associaton
185. Holoprosencephaly (single case)

Some Other Facts About the Syndrome:
• Population prevalence (estimated): 1:2,000 people
• Birth incidence (estimated): 1:1,800 births
• Prevalence in infants with conotruncal heart anomalies: 10% to 30%
• Prevalence in cleft palate (without cleft lip): 8%

Feeding in VCFS

The neonatal period of babies with VCFS is often medically stormy, complicated by cardiac problems, immunodeficiency, hypocalcemia, and hypotonicity. Facial asymmetry during crying is a frequent finding. With or without cleft palate, feeding problems and failure to thrive are common, resulting in referrals to SLPs for feeding therapy. Feeding may be complicated by generalized and pharyngeal hypotonia, laryngeal anomalies, or vascular anomalies, such as vascular rings that could compress the pharyngeal structures. Nasal regurgitation and nasal vomiting are frequent. Feeding may be further complicated by airway obstruction that could result from Robin sequence and/or pharyngeal hypotonia.

Many infants with VCFS establish functional feeding skills using the modifications described in Chapter 4. The baby should be held in as upright a position as possible and the nipple opening should be enlarged slightly by making a cross-cut. Feeding schedules may also need to be modified because the generalized hypotonia associated with VCFS causes the stomach and gut to clear slowly, so that putting more food into an already full stomach may induce vomiting. Although many patients with VCFS have been treated with gastrostomies and nasogastric tubes, such drastic strategies are rarely required. The use of oral stimulation techniques that are often recommended in other patients are typically not effective in VCFS because feeding problems are frequently a combination of hypotonia, heart disease, respiratory disorder, slow clearing of the digestive tract, and temperament.

Speech and Language in VCFS

Speech and language characteristics of VCFS include receptive and expressive language delays, hypernasality that is usually severe, a severe articulation disorder characterized by compensatory errors, primarily glottal stops, high pitched voice, and hoarseness (Golding-Kushner et al., 1985; Golding-Kushner, 1991; Scherer et al., 1999; Shprintzen, 2000; D'Antonio et al., 2000). Physiological anomalies leading to the resonance and voice problems include anterior laryngeal web and velopharyngeal insufficiency that is usually severe (Golding-Kushner, 1991; Lipson, 1995; Shprintzen, 2000). Dyspraxia or apraxia are frequently diagnosed but are almost always a misdiagnosis.

Speech and language delays in VCFS are usually apparent from the onset of language (Shprintzen et al., 1978; Golding-Kushner et al., 1985; Scherer et al., 1999). Expressive language and speech skills tend to be disproportionately low in comparison to the receptive language delay (Scherer et al., 1999; D'Antonio et al., 2000). Therefore, babies with VCFS should receive aggressive early intervention services to stimulate oral language development.

Children with VCFS learn differently from other children with cleft palate, so the clinician and parents must adjust their expectations accordingly. Even if it appears that the child is not responding, they must continue stimulating speech and language. Improvement may take a long time but will occur. The learning curve of children with VCFS may be more stepwise than smooth, and it is important not to become discouraged by the plateaus. Some children with VCFS remain relatively nonverbal until age $2\frac{1}{2}$ or 3 years (Scherer et al., 1999). Some children with VCFS seem to demonstrate a period of rapid catch-up in the late preschool through early school age period (D'Antonio et al., 2000). One of the learning characteristics of children with VCFS is that their ability to learn and retain information on a single presentation is limited. Therefore, sessions should be frequent and short, in order to provide maximum repetition. If frequent sessions (three to five times per week) are not possible, the sessions may be longer, but a break should be taken after 10 minutes. Treatment may then be resumed for another segment of the allotted time.

Some personality characteristics associated with VCFS must also be considered in planning intervention. Children with VCFS tend to startle easily, may be phobic, and may have tactile defensiveness. These may be early symptoms of the psychiatric disorders that tend to manifest in later childhood or during the teenage years. They should not be assumed to be reflective of a sensory integration disorder. Because of these characteristics, infants and young children with VCFS should be approached gently. The clinician should ease herself/himself into the child's "space" and be careful to integrate the parent into the session activities to help the child feel safe. It is even more effective to begin play with the parent and then allow the child to join the activity. Home programs are especially advantageous for babies with VCFS who may have difficulty coping with changes in environment.

Even as they develop conversational skills, expressive language may appear uneven and cyclic, possibly reflecting early manifestations of psychiatric disease often diagnosed in adolescence and early adulthood. For example, during a behavioral cycle in which they are shy and withdrawn, they may produce one- or two-word sentences. The same child may then go through a cycle during which their behavior is more animated and they speak constantly. These cycles are unpredictable and may last for hours or weeks. SLPs working with children with VCFS should be aware of these behavioral issues and adjust the procedures for therapy sessions (not the goals) accordingly.

Some clinicians advocate the use of total communication programs as a "bridge" with very young children with VCFS who are nonverbal, making sure that the emphasis remains on oral communication (Scherer & D'Antonio, 1998). On the other hand, Golding-Kushner and Shprintzen (1998) point out that the additional goal of teaching signs to a normally hearing child with normal speech potential who is already delayed in speech and language places an unnecessary additional therapeutic burden on everyone involved in the process, and distracts the clinician, parent, and child from the business of learning to speak. It is like asking a child to learn two foreign languages, their cultural language, such as English or Spanish, and sign language. This is a great demand to place on a child struggling as he or she is to learn even one language.

VCFS and Speech and Language Therapy at School

Most children with VCFS receive speech and language services at school. In fact, there are probably many children on the caseloads of school SLPs who have VCFS but have not been diagnosed. VCFS should be suspected in any child with learning disability and "cleft palate speech," even if a cleft palate is not known to be present. Children with cleft palate and speech problems, and children with VCFS in particular, may pose several challenges for school-based SLPs. Children typically receive speech services at school in groups as large as five students, for sessions ranging from 15 to 30 minutes. This is simply not effective for children with VCFS, most of whom require both articulation and language therapy. As stated above, children with VCFS learn best in frequent, short sessions with a lot of repetition.

Treatment goals for children with VCFS must be prioritized, taking into account other medical, social, and educational issues. The needs may be divided into speech and language domains. The speech needs include articulation therapy to eliminate glottal stops, and pharyngeal surgery to eliminate VPI and hypernasality. The language needs include therapy to improve receptive and expressive skills, and skills related to abstract thinking and social communication. In terms of prioritization, the child must have sufficient language to allow analysis and treatment of the articulation errors. Hypernasality cannot be diagnosed adequately in nonverbal or in minimally verbal children. Thus, language therapy should be the priority for a minimally verbal child. Articulation therapy may be integrated into the language focus by centering therapy on functional words and concepts likely to elicit production of phonemes in the sequence outlined in the precious chapters.

Once the child is producing two and three word phrases, there is usually a sufficient amount of speech to analyze resonance. When significant hypernasality is present, the clinician should refer the child with VCFS back to the cleft palate team for decisions about management of VPI. If resonance is severely hypernasal, as is usually the case in VCFS, pharyngoplasty should be considered. In most children with glottal stops and hypernasality, the recommendation is to eliminate the glottal stops first and to plan pharyngeal surgery after speech therapy has been successful in doing so. This is because many speakers demonstrate improved velopharyngeal movements when they produce correct, oral articulation rather than during the production of glottal stops (Golding, 1981; Henningsson et al., 1986; Golding-Kushner, 1989, 1995; Shprintzen, 1990; Ysunza, 1992). This is not the case among children with VCFS. Their pharyngeal movements tend to be hypotonic and deficient even when they produce correct oral articulation (Golding-Kushner, 1995). Velopharyngeal movements also tend not to improve in most children with VCFS after use of a speech bulb appliance, even though articulation does improve (Golding-Kushner et al., 1995). This is probably because of the many factors that contribute to VPI in VCFS, including thin pharyngeal tissue (Golding-Kushner, 1991), adenoid hypoplasia (Arvystas & Shprintzen, 1984), and vascular anomalies (Mitnick et al., 1996). Furthermore, some individuals with VCFS appear to establish velopharyngel closure on sustained fricatives /s, f/ or during production of single words, but do not sustain closure during connected speech. Their closure appears to "pulse" open and closed. For all these reasons, it is recommended that children with VCFS undergo physical management of their VPI as soon as it can be examined adequately, usually by age 4 years. Following pharyngoplasty, the treatment priority should shift to articulation. This is because articulation therapy can be accomplished more quickly than language therapy, which tends to be more protracted with needs for increased complexity evolving over time. In contrast, articulation therapy involves a finite number of phonemes and has a clear end point. The goal of normal speech production is realistic and achievable in a relatively short time. Abnormal speech is one of the disorders associated with VCFS that can be treated and eliminated as a problem. Speech therapy does not occur without language. Therefore, the statement that the treatment priority should shift to articulation is not meant to imply that language is being ignored. However, during that period of therapy, which may last from 6 to 12 months, the language goals should be integrated into articulation drill therapy. When abnormal compensatory errors are eliminated, the articulation goals related to carryover should be integrated into the language therapy. As stated earlier, it is the current trend to view articulation and language as a single entity. However, that approach has proven to be less effective in the treatment of compensatory speech errors than the approach advocated in this book. This is especially true as applied to the treatment of speech disorders in children with VCFS.

To be most effective, speech therapy to eliminate glottal stops should be scheduled three to five times per week for 20 to 30 minutes on an individual basis. Again, the emphasis on minimum number of correct productions each session may necessitate a *temporary* emphasis on articulation with language goals considered secondary. The techniques to eliminate glottal stops in children with VCFS is the same as for other children. The need for frequent, intensive sessions and daily home practice are even more important because of their reliance on repetition as an important learning tool.

As the child with VCFS moves to the sentence level of treatment, higher, increasing integration of language goals is possible. Language therapy should provide emphasis on development of abstract reasoning skills as well as pragmatic skills. Social language is an area of concern for many children and adolescents with VCFS. When their articulation errors have been corrected, it may be appropriate to shift from individual to small group therapy for some of the sessions so that pragmatic skills can be improved in a realistic social context. If other language goals remain, some therapy should continue on an individual basis because of the fact that children with VCFS benefit from 1:1 teaching and repetition. In this situation, consideration should be given to scheduling individual therapy two to three times per week in addition to one to two group sessions.

VCFS and Learning

Most children with VCFS are of normal or borderline normal intelligence, although some are mildly mentally retarded. Learning disabilities are common, most often affecting reading comprehension and math concepts, and tasks involving inferential reasoning and abstract thinking are especially difficult (Golding-Kushner et al., 1985). Therefore, learning disabilities in some children with VCFS may not manifest until second or third grade, when academic demands are greater and learning is increasingly dependent on reading and auditory processing of complex material. The learning style in children with VCFS tends to show alternating patterns of plateaus and leaps, during which skills drilled during the preceding plateau emerge. This is especially evident during the language learning of the first 3 years of life.

School performance is also affected by ADHD, another frequent finding in VCFS. Children with VCFS may do relatively well in the early school years. However, as school learning depends increasingly on reading comprehension and material becomes more abstract and complex, performance tends to drop. Children with VCFS tend to rely on concrete thinking processes, making the increasingly abstract material very difficult. They also may have psychological characteristics affecting behavior that may affect learning. Many children with VCFS are very shy and, even when capable of more, avoid verbal interaction, limiting their responses in the classroom to single or two word phrases. One of the psychiatric disorders associated with VCFS in teenagers and adults is bipolar disorder which is characterized by periods of withdrawal and periods of mania (Papolos et al., 1996). Therefore, verbal responses among affected individuals may be terse at times and verbose at others. Another characteristic is impulsivity, which affects classroom and social functioning (Golding-Kushner et al., 1985). They may have trouble with transitions, making it difficult for them to change activities within the classroom, and even more difficult to move between classrooms to go to a resource or speech therapy room. They may need assistance to get used to going to various rooms, and time to adjust to the change once there. The use of FM units in the classroom may be helpful to improve focusing.

OTHER SYNDROMES

VCFS is only one of over 400 identified syndromes that may be associated with cleft palate and/or VPI. Many of these syndromes are relatively common and have patterns of communication development and disorders that have been documented in at least some cases, sometimes in large numbers of cases. *Stickler syndrome* is a genetic disorder affecting the connective tissue, and affected individuals may have incomplete cleft palate or submucous cleft palate, severe, progressive myopia (nearsightedness), and early arthritis (Jones, 1988; Gorlin et al., 1990). If undiagnosed, young children may complain of painful joints that are dismissed as "growing pains." High frequency sensorineural hearing loss and scoliosis are other findings. Airway obstruction related to Robin sequence is common in infancy and it has been estimated that one-third of all cases of Robin sequence actually have Stickler syndrome (Shprintzen, 1992). About half of children with Stickler syndrome who have cleft palate develop normal speech and resonance, and about half of them are hypernasal and have compensatory articulation disorders (Golding-Kushner, 1991). Their hypernasality, when present, tends to be mild. Language and learning skills are usually normal, especially when hearing is normal and middle ear disease associated with cleft palate is treated vigilantly (Golding-Kushner, 1991). As can be seen, the prognosis for children with Stickler syndrome is quite different from that of children with VCFS. If medical care is vigilant, especially otologic, they are at low risk for language and learning problems and hypernasality, if present, can be expected to be mild.

Another genetic syndrome of interest to speech pathologists is *Treacher Collins syndrome,* which affects the face, orbits, and ears bilaterally. Cleft palate and submucous cleft palate occur frequently. Maximum conductive hearing loss secondary to outer and middle ear malformations is common, and is the greatest threat to cognitive, speech, and language development, especially if not detected and treated early. Because of bilateral microtia and/or atresia, use of a bone conduction hearing aid may be necessary. The vocal tract is extremely narrow in Treacher Collins syndrome, and airway obstruction is very common in infancy (Shprintzen et al., 1979). Following palate repair, nasal resonance is usually normal. Hypernasality, when it occurs, tends to be very mild or intermittent and may decrease or even resolve with age because of changes in the nasopharynx and vocal tract that occur as a result of craniofacial growth patterns (Golding-Kushner, 1991). Articulation errors tend to involve tongue backing, and compensatory errors related to VPI are infrequent (Golding-Kushner, 1991). Oral resonance may be muffled because the oral cavity and vocal tract are small. The observation that resonance tends to improve with growth distinguishes this syndrome from others associated with cleft palate and VPI, and is of obvious significance in avoiding potentially unnecessary surgery.

Information about speech, language, voice, and resonance in specific syndromes is becoming increasingly available both in print and on-line. One such recent publication includes brief descriptions of communication aspects and other features of 160 syndromes (Shprintzen, 2000).

OTHER SPECIAL GROUPS

Many children have unusual oral anomalies that are not part of a recognized syndrome. The principles and techniques that have been described may be applied to their treatment as well. It is essential to evaluate speech sound and language development at the earliest possible opportunity, and to provide parent training and early intervention as necessary. The clinician must differentiate between speech errors that are obligatory in the presence of a particular child's oral architecture, and those that are not obligatory, keeping in mind that most articulation errors are *not* obligatory. The child seen in Figure 10–2 was born with an unusual pattern of severe oral anomalies that may have been related to a crowded intrauterine position as a twin. Although his twin brother was born with a normal mouth and jaw, this child was born with an underdeveloped mandible that was fused to the maxilla on the left, an incomplete and asymmetric cleft palate, and microglossia. The lingual tissue that was present was contiguous with the buccal (cheek) surface on the left, restricting movement of the free right lateral margin and tip, and there were mounds of excess tissue on the superior lingual surface. The importance of distinguishing between obligatory and compensatory errors is illustrated by his case history.

Case History

The patient seen in Figure 10–2, G., was referred for early intervention services for feeding and speech at about 8 months of age, with tracheotomy and feeding gastrostomy tubes in place. He had received no oral feedings and had undergone no reconstructive surgery. He lived at home with his parents, his twin, and an older brother, but was cared for during the day by a team of nurses because both parents were employed full time out of the home. Within a few months, he was on full oral feeding and a Passy Muir valve was fit on his trach so that sound production was possible. He began producing nasal consonants and vowels. Shortly thereafter, he was decannulated and the feeding tube was removed. Because he was doing so well medically, full-time nursing services were discontinued by his insurance company and he began attending day care on a full-time basis. Scheduling conflicts necessitated that a different clinician assume his speech therapy, and he was not seen by the author for several years. According to his parents, G. received limited speech therapy during that time, and the clinicians that saw him told the parents that he was doing as well as could be expected until his palate was repaired. The parents had been told that

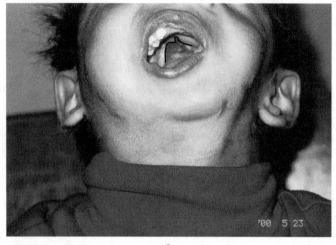

A

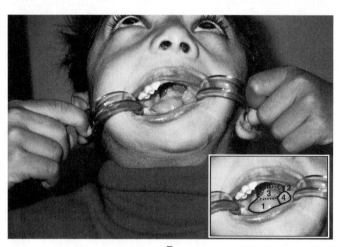

B

FIGURE 10-2. Child with oral anomalies probably related to intrauterine position and crowding. Oral opening achieved following surgical creation of a TMJ. (**A**) Note unusual shape of cleft palate with intact lateral shelf on right, irregular anterior edge and width of defect on left. Primary dentition is limited to a few teeth on the right maxillary and mandibular arches. (**B**) Lingual anomalies. (**1**) The top and right lateral edge appear normal, (**2**) Note contiguity of left side of tongue with buccal tissue, (**3**) mounds on dorsal surface of the tongue, (**4**) and excess mound of tissue at junction of tongue and cheek on left.

the likelihood of normal speech was slim, given the severity of his anomalies, and that consideration should be given to an augmentative communication device, which they resisted. The assumption that his speech errors were obligatory in the presence of his abnormal oral structure was a major error that resulted in significant loss of valuable therapy time.

G. was referred back to the author at age 5 years, following surgery to create a temporomandibular joint on the right by insertion of a metal ball. He was referred for exercises to maintain the oral opening that was achieved in surgery and for feeding therapy. Although he had been eating soft foods adequately prior to surgery, he was having difficulty postoperatively with all consistencies. It was interesting and very distressing that he was not referred for speech therapy, because, in spite of completely normal language skills, he exhibited a profound speech disorder, characterized by exclusive production of glottal stops and neutral vowels. He did not move his lips (which were unaffected by his oral anomalies) at all during speech, and was not even producing the /m/ he had babbled at age 1 year. Lack of movement of the tongue, the left surface of which adhered to the right cheek, together with lack of jaw and lip movement resulted in the limited repertoire of distorted, neutral vowels. On request, he was able to move the dorsum, free right edge, and tip of his tongue. The palate had not yet been repaired because his oral opening was still too limited to allow surgeons access to the palate. Because of his still limited oral opening and severely restricted tongue movement, it would have been easy to once again dismiss many of his speech errors as obligatory.

After consultation with the cleft palate team and insurance company, G. began a coordinated program of speech therapy that included private therapy three times per week for 1 hour each, school-based therapy two times per week on an individual basis for 30 minutes each session, and a daily program of home practice. The private therapy was of 1-hour duration to allow time to establish chewing skills that had not been possible prior to creation of the TMJ, and to perform oral manipulation requested by the maxillofacial surgeon to maintain opening of the jaw. At least 30 minutes of each session was devoted to articulation therapy, using the articulation therapy techniques described in this manual. Within 10 months, G. established correct deliberate (but not automatic) production in structured phrases and sentences of all vowels and diphthongs, semivowels, nasals /m, n, ŋ/, plosives /p, b, t, d, k, g/, and fricatives /f, v, θ/. He also established oral production of sibilants /s, z, ʃ/ in imitation in syllables. His progress was evidence that G.'s speech errors were compensatory, not obligatory. In spite of limited tongue mobility, 5 years of lack of use of the lips, jaw, and tongue for speech, the presence of an open cleft palate, and the presence of only a few teeth on the left side of the mouth, he learned production of all these sounds. It should be emphasized that "oral-motor" exercises were *not* used to increase lip or tongue strength or mobility. Use of the lips and tongue was elicited by teaching, demonstrating and reinforcing their correct movement during sound production. Every time the target sounds were produced, use of the lips and/or tongue improved. For example, lip rounding for /u/ and /w/ were elicited by the reminder, "pointy lips." The phonemes targeted and the sequence in which they were introduced are listed in Table 10–2.

After 10 months, speech production was significantly improved when the nostrils were occluded, confirming that persistent weak intraoral pressure, nasal emission and turbulence, and hypernasality were obligatory. G. returned to the treating cleft palate team who were pleasantly surprised by his speech progress, and determined that he had maintained sufficient oral opening to allow surgeons to proceed with an attempt to repair his palate. Because the cleft was so wide and the tissue in the surrounding area so limited, the team decided that a primary pharyngeal flap would be necessary. This would increase the risk of airway obstruction, and raised the possibility that a tracheotomy would, again, be necessary. Prosthetic management was not possible because of the limited oral opening and lack of dentition and supporting tissue for retention of an appliance. The parents weighed their options and decided to proceed with surgery to facilitate speech, even if it meant another period of time with a trach and Passy-Muir speaking valve. G. is currently awaiting a date for surgery while continuing to work on increasing consistency and automaticity of use of correct articulation, and learning to produce sibilant sounds. The insurance company is "deciding" if they will continue to cover his private therapy.

Feeding therapy has been discontinued. G.'s eating skills are completely functional in terms of nutrition and weight gain using his limited "munch" bite, and he eats a regular diet, in spite of his inability to produce a "normal" rotary chew or to use his tongue to push food on to the left side of his mouth which is where his few teeth are.

TABLE 10-2 *Sequence in Which Target Phonemes Were Introduced to G.*

Dates are included to provide a timing reference. Sounds on the same line were introduced during the same session.

Start 9/14:	/h/
	/u/
	/u/ → /a/ ("oooah") to elicit /w/
	/m/
	/e, o, i, ɛ, a, æ/
	/p/
	/ɚ/ (emerged spontaneously), r
	/aɪ/ (as in eye), ɔ
	/n, l/
	/b/
	/j/
	/t, d/
11/5:	phrases: a _____, no _____,
	phrases: I want _____, I have _____
11/19:	/f/
12/20:	/ŋ, k/
	/ɔɪ/
	r-vowels
2/3:	/g/
4/7:	/θ/
4/17:	/ð/ /s/

REFERENCES

Arvystas, M., & Shprintzen R.J. (1984). Craniofacial morphology in velo-cardio-facial syndrome. *Journal of Craniofacial Genetics and Developmental Biology, 4* (1), 39–45.

Bardach J., & Morris H.L (Eds.). (1990). *Multidisciplinary management of cleft lip and palate,* Philadelphia, PA: Saunders.

Borden, G.J., & Harris K.S. (1980). *Speech science primer: Physiology, acoustics and perception of speech.* Baltimore, MD: Williams and Wilkins.

Chapman, K. (1993). Phonologic processes in children with cleft palate. *Cleft Palate Craniofacial Journal, 30,* 64–71.

D'Antonio, L.L., & Scherer, N.J. (1995). The evaluation of speech disorders associated with clefting. In R.J. Shprintzen & J. Bardach (Eds.), *Cleft palate speech management: A multidisciplinary approach* (pp. 176–220). St. Louis, MO: Mosby.

D'Antonio, L.L., Scherer, N.J., Miller L.L., Kalbfleisch, J.H., & Bartley J.A. (in press). Analysis of speech characteristics in children with velocardiofacial syndrome and children with phenotypic overlap without VCFS. *Cleft Palate Journal.*

Duffy, J.R. (1995). *Motor speech disorders: Substrates, differential diagnosis and management.* St. Louis, MO: Mosby Year Book, Inc.

Fenson, L., Dale, P.S., Reznick, J.S., Thal, D., Bates, E., Hartung, J.P., Pethick, S., & Reilly, J.S. (1991). *The MacArthur communicative development inventory: Toddlers.* San Diego, CA: Singular Publishing Group.

Fudala, J.B. (2000). *Arizona 3.* Los Angeles, CA: Western Psychological Services.

Golding, K.J. (1981). *Articulation and velopharyngeal insufficiency: A rationale for pre-surgical speech therapy.* Fourth International Congress on Cleft Palate and Related Craniofacial Anomalies, Acapulco, Mexico.

Golding, K.J., & Kaslon, K. (1981). A home program for infant stimulation. *Annual Symposium of the Center for Craniofacial Disorders of Montefiore Hospital and Medical Center and the Albert Einstein College of Medicine.* Bronx, NY.

Golding-Kushner, K.J. (1989). *Speech therapy for compensatory articulation errors in patients with "cleft palate speech."* Videotape produced by the Center for Craniofacial Disorders, Montefiore Medical Center, Bronx, NY.

Golding-Kushner, K.J. (1991). *Craniofacial morphology and velopharyngeal physiology in four syndromes of clefting.* Unpublished doctoral dissertation, The Graduate School and University Center, City University of NY.

Golding-Kushner, K.J. (1995). Treatment of articulation and resonance disorders associated with cleft palate and VPI. In R.J. Shprintzen & J. Bardach (Eds.), *Cleft palate speech management: A multidisciplinary approach.* (pp. 327–351). St. Louis, MO: Mosby.

Golding-Kushner, K.J. (1997). Cleft lip and palate, craniofacial anomalies and velopharyngeal insufficiency. In C. Ferrand & R. Bloom, (Eds), *Introduction to neurogenic and organic disorders of communication: Current scope of practice,* (pp. 193–228). Boston, MA: Allyn and Bacon.

Golding-Kushner K.J., Argamaso, R.V., Cotton, R.T., Grames, L.M., Henningsson, G., Jones, D.L., Karnell, M.P., Klaiman, P.G., Lewin, M.L., Marsh, J.L., McCall, G.N., McGrath, C.O., Muntz, H.R., Nevdahl, M.T., Rakoff, S.J., Shprintzen, S.J., Sidoti, E.J., Vallino, L.D., Volk, M., Williams, W.N., Witzel, M.A., Wood, V.D., Ysunza, A., D'Antonio, L.L., Isberg, A., Pigott, R.W., Skolnick, M.L. (1990). Standardization for the reporting of nasopharyngoscopy and multiview videofluoroscopy: A report from an International Working Group. *Cleft Palate Journal, 27* (4), 337–347.

Golding-Kushner K.J., Cisneros G., and LeBlanc, E. (1995). Speech bulbs. In R.J. Shprintzen & J. Bardach (Eds.), *Cleft palate speech management: A multidisciplinary approach* (pp. 352–363). St. Louis, MO: Mosby.

Golding-Kushner, K.J., LeBlanc, S., & Tantillo, M. (1990). *The speech therapy team: Redefining the concept.* Miniseminar. American Speech and Hearing Association, Seattle, WA.

Golding-Kushner, K.J. & Shprintzen R.J. (1998). To sign or not to sign: Con. *VCFSEF Newsletter.* Syracuse, NY: VCFS Educational Foundation.

Golding-Kushner, K.J., Weller, G., & Shprintzen, R.J. (1985). Velocardio-facial syndrome: Language and psychological characteristics. *Journal of Craniofacial Genetics and Developmental Biology, 5* (3), 259–266.

Gorlin, R.J., Cohen, M.M., Levin, L.S. (1990). *Syndromes of the head and neck* (3rd ed.). New York: Oxford University Press.

Hall, C., & Golding-Kushner, K.J. (1989) *Long-term follow-up of 500 patients after palate repair performed prior to 18 months of age.* Paper presented at the Sixth International Congress on Cleft Palate and Related Craniofacial Anomalies, Jerusalem, Israel.

Harding-Bell, A. (2000). *Multiple Objective Input Therapy: A model for ad-dressing several aspects of communicative behavior.* Annual Meeting of the Velo-cardio-facial Syndrome Educational Foundation. Balti-more, MD.

Hedrick, D.L., Prather, E.M., & Tobin, A.R. (1984). *Sequenced inventory of communicative development.* Seattle, WA: University of Washington Press.

Henningsson, G.E., & Isberg, A.M. (1986). Velopharyngeal movements in patients alternating between oral and glottal articulation: a clin-ical and cineradiographical study. *Cleft Palate Journal, 23*, 1–9.

Hoch, L., Golding-Kushner, K.J., Sadewitz, V., & Shprintzen, R.J. (1986). Speech therapy. In B.J. McWilliams (Ed.). *Seminars in speech and lan-guage: Current methods of assessing and treating children with cleft palates, 7* (3), 313–326. New York: Thieme.

Isberg, A.M., & Henningsson, G.E. (1987). Influence of palatal fistulas on velopharyngeal movements: A cineradiographic study. *Plastic and Reconstructive Surgery, 79*, 525–530.

Johns, D.F. (1985). Surgical and prosthetic management of neurogenic velopharyngeal incompetence. In D.F. Johns (Ed.), *Clinical manage-ment of communicative disorders,* Boston, MA: Little Brown. (pp. 153–178).

Jones, K.L. (1988). *Smith's recognizable patterns of human malformation.* Philadelphia, PA: W.B. Saunders.

Kok, L.K., & Solman, R.T. (1995). Velocardiofacial syndrome: learn-ing difficulties and intervention. *Journal of Medical Genetics, 32*, 612–618.

Kuehn, D.P., & Moon, J.B. (1994). Levator veli palatini muscle activity in relation to intraoral air pressure variation. *Journal of Speech and Hearing Research, 37* (6), 1260–70.

Lipson, A. (1995). *The changing phenotype and extraordinary variability of VCF: 200 cases from down under.* Paper presented at the First Annual Meeting of the Velo-cardio-facial Syndrome Educational Founda-tion, Bronx, NY.

Lynch, J.I. (1986). Language of cleft infants: Lessening the risk of delay through programming. In B.J. McWilliams (Ed.), *Seminars in speech and language: Current methods of assessing and treating children with cleft palates, 7* (3), 255–268. New York: Thieme.

McGrath, C.O., & Anderson, M.W. (1990). Prosthetic treatment of velopharyngeal incompetence. In J. Bardach & H.L. Morris (Eds.), *Multidisciplinary management of cleft lip and palate* (pp. 809–815). Philadelphia, PA: W.B. Saunders.

McWilliams, B.J., Morris, H.L., & Shelton R.L. (1990). *Cleft palate speech* (2nd ed.). Philadelphia, PA: B.C. Decker.

Mitnick, R.J, Bello, J.A., Golding-Kushner, K.J., Argamaso, R.V., Shprintzen, R.J. (1996). The use of magnetic resonance angiography prior to pharyngeal flap surgery in patients with velocardiofacial syndrome. *Plastic and Reconstructive Surgery, 97,* 908–919.

Morley, M.E. (1970). *Cleft palate and speech.* (7th ed.) Baltimore, MD: Williams and Wilkins.

Morley, M.E. (1972). *The development and disorders of speech in childhood* (3rd ed.). Baltimore, MD: Williams and Wilkins.

Pamplona, M., & Ysunza, A. (1999a). A comparitive trial of two modalities of speech intervention in cleft palate children: Phonologic vs. articulatory approach. *International Journal of Pediatric Otorhinolaryngology, 49,* 21–27.

Pamplona, M., & Ysunza, A. (1999b). Active participation of mothers during speech therapy: Improved language development of children with cleft palate. *Scandinavian Journal of Plastic Reconstructive Hand Surgery, 33:* 1–6.

Pamplona, M., Ysunza A., & Uriostegui, C. (1996). Linguistic interaction: The active role of parents in speech therapy for cleft palate patients. *International Journal of Pediatric Otorhinolaryngology, 37:* 17–27.

Papolos, D.F., Faedda, G.L., Veit, S., Goldberg, R., Morrow, B., Kucherlapati R., Shprintzen, R.J. (1996). Bipolar spectrum disorders in patients diagnosed with velo-cardio-facial syndrome: Does a hemizygous deletion of chromosome 22q11 result in bipolar affective disorder? *American Journal of Psychiatry, 153,* 1541–1547.

Peterson-Falzone, S. (1990). A cross-sectional analysis of speech results following palatal closure. In J. Bardach & H.L. Morris (Eds.), *Multidisciplinary management of cleft lip and palate* (pp 750–757). Philadelphia, PA: W.B. Saunders.

Phillips, B.J. (1990). Early speech management. In J. Bardach & H.L. Morris (Eds.), *Multidisciplinary management of cleft lip and palate* (pp 732–736). Philadelphia, W.B. Saunders Company.

Philips, B.J., & Kent, R.D. (1984). Acoustic-phonetic descriptions of speech production in speakers with cleft palate and other velopharyngeal disorders. In N. Lass (Ed.) *Speech and language: Advances in basic research and practice.* (Vol. 11, p. 113) New York: Academic Press.

Powers, G. (1990). Speech analysis of four children with repaired cleft palate. *Journal of Speech and Hearing Disorders, 55,* 542–550.

Powers, G., & Starr C.D. (1974). The effects of muscle exercises on velopharyngeal gap and nasality. *Cleft Palate Journal, 11,* 28–35.

Richman, L.C., & Eliason, M.J. (1986). Development in children with cleft lip and/or palate: Intellectual, cognitive, personality and parental factors. In B.J. McWilliams (Ed.), *Seminars in speech and language: Current methods of assessing and treating children with cleft palates, 7* (3), 225–239. New York: Thieme.

Robin, D.A., Solomon, N.P., Moon, J., & Folkins J.W. (1997). Non-speech assessment of the speech production mechanism. In McNeil, M.R. (Ed), *Clinical management of sensorimotor speech disorders.* (pp. 49–62). New York: Thieme.

Rossetti, L. (1990). *Infant-Toddler Language Scale.* East Moline, IL: Linguisystems.

Ruscello, D.M. (1982). A selected review of palatal training procedures. *Cleft Palate Journal, 18,* 181–193.

Scherer, N.J., & D'Antonio, L.L. (1995). Parent questionnaire for screening early language development in children with cleft palate. *Cleft Palate—Craniofacial Journal. 32* (1), 7–12.

Scherer, N.J., & D'Antonio, L.L. (1997). Language and play development in toddlers with cleft lip and/or palate. *American Journal of Speech-Language Pathology, 6* (4), 48–54.

Scherer, N.J., and D'Antonio L.L. (1998). To sign or not to sign: Pro. *VCFSEF Newsletter.* Syracuse, NY: VCFS Educational Foundation.

Scherer, N.J., D'Antonio, L.L., & Kalbfleisch, J.H. (1999). Early speech and language development in children with velocardiofacial syndrome. *American Journal of Medical Genetics (Neuropsychiatric Genetics), 88,* 714–723.

Shprintzen, R.J. (1990). The conceptual framework for pharyngeal flap surgery. In J. Bardach & H.L. Morris (Eds.), *Multidisciplinary management of cleft lip and palate* (pp. 806–809). Philadelphia, PA: W.B. Saunders.

Shprintzen, R.J. (1992). The implications of the diagnosis of Robin sequence. *Cleft Palate Journal, 29,* 205–209.

Shprintzen, R.J. (2000). *Syndrome identification for speech-language pathology: An illustrated pocket guide.* San Diego, CA: Singular Publishing Group.

Shprintzen, R.J., & Bardach, J. (Eds.) (1990). *Cleft palate speech management: A multidisciplinary approach.* St. Louis, MO: Mosby.

Shprintzen, R.J., Croft, C.B., Berkman, M.D., & Rakoff, S.J. (1979). Pharyngeal hypoplasia in Treacher Collins syndrome. *Archives of Otolaryngology, 105* (3) 127–131.

Shprintzen, R.J., Goldberg, R.B., Lewin, M.L., Sidoti, E.J., Berkman, M.D., Argamaso, R.V., & Young, D. (1978). A new syndrome involving cleft palate, cardiac anomalies, typical facies, and learning disabilities: Velo-cardio-facial syndrome. *Cleft Palate Journal, 15* (1), 56–62.

Shprintzen, R.J., & Golding-Kushner, K.J. (1989). Evaluation of velopharyngeal insufficiency. In G. Healy & E. Friedman (Eds.), *Otolaryngologic clinics of North America, 22,* (3) 519–536. Philadelphia, PA: W.B. Saunders.

Shprintzen, R.J., McCall, G., & Skolnick, M.L. (1975). A new therapeutic technique for the treatment of velopharyngeal incompetence. *Journal of Speech and Hearing Disorders, 40,* 69–83.

Sidoti, E.J., & Shprintzen, R.J. (1995). Pediatric care and feeding of the newborn with a cleft. In R.J. Shprintzen, & J. Bardach (Eds.), *Cleft palate speech management: A multidisciplinary approach* (pp. 63–74). St. Louis, MO: Mosby.

Singh, S., & Kent, R.D. (2000) *Singular's Illustrated Dictionary of Speech-Language Pathology;* San Diego, CA: Singular Publishing Group.

Specialist Fact Sheet (2000) [On-line]. The Velo-Cardio-Facial Syndrome Educational Foundation, Inc. Web site. http://www.vcfsef. org/.

Starr, C.D. (1990). Treatment by therapeutic exercises. In J. Bardach, & H.L. Morris (Eds.), *Multidisciplinary management of cleft lip and palate* (pp. 792–798). Philadelphia, PA: W.B. Saunders.

Stedman's medical dictionary (1976). Baltimore, MD: Williams and Wilkins.

Trigos, I., Ysunza, A., Vargas, D., & Vazquez, M. (1988). The San Venero Roselli pharyngoplasty: An electromyographic study of the palatopharyngeus muscle. *Cleft Palate Journal, 25,* 385–388.

Trost, J. (1981). Articulatory additions to the classical description of the speech of persons with cleft palate. *Cleft Palate Journal 18,* (3), 193–203.

Van Demark, D.R., & Hardin, M.A. (1990). Speech therapy for the child with cleft lip and palate. In J. Bardach, & H.L. Morris (Eds.), *Multidisciplinary management of cleft lip and palate* (pp. 799–806). Philadelphia, PA: W.B. Saunders,

Van Hattum, R.J. (1974) *Clinical speech in the schools: organization and management.* Springfield, IL: Charles C. Thomas.

Van Riper, C. (1972). *Speech correction: Principles and methods.* Englewood Cliffs, NJ: Prentice-Hall.

Warren, D.W. (1986). Compensatory speech behaviors in cleft palate: A regulation control phenomenon? *Cleft Palate Journal, 23,* 251–260.

Ysunza, A., Pamplona, M., Chason, E., et al. (1999). Velopharyngeal motion following pharyngoplasty. *Plastic and Reconstructive Surgery, 104,* 905–910.

Ysunza, A., Pamplona, M., Mayer, I., et al. (1996). Surgical correction of VPI with and without compensatory articulation. *International Journal of Pediatric Otorhinolaryngology, 34,* 53–59.

Ysunza, A., Pamplona, C., & Toledo, E. (1992). Change in velopharyngeal valving after speech therapy in cleft palate patients: A video-nasopharyngoscopic and multi-view videofluoroscopic study. *International Journal of Pediatric Otorhinolaryngoly, 24,* 45–54.

Zimmerman, I.R., Steiner, V.G., & Pond, R.E. (1992). *Pre-school language scale-3.* San Antonio, TX: Psychological Corporation.

A P P E N D I X

Resources for Parents and Professionals

American Cleft Palate-Craniofacial Association (ACPA)
ACPA National Office
104 South Estes Drive, Suite 204
Chapel Hill, NC 27514
(Tel) (919) 933-9044
(Fax) (919) 933-9604
Website: www.cleft.com
email: cleftline@aol.com

American Speech-Language Hearing Association (ASHA)
10801 Rockville Pike
Rockville, Maryland 20852
(Tel) 800-498-2071
(TTY) 301-897-5700
(Fax) 301-571-0457
Website: www.asha.org (This web site includes information on IDEA) also,
Special Interest Division 5, "Speech Science and Orofacial Disorders"

Velo-cardio-facial Syndrome Educational Foundation, Inc. (VCFSEF)
Upstate Medical University
University Hospital
750 East Adams Street
Syracuse, NY 13210
(Tel) (315) 464-6590
(Fax) (315) 464- 6593
Website: www.vcfsef.org
email: vcfsef@mail.upstate.edu

For referrals to speech centers or private SLPs:
Contact the Speech-Language Hearing Association in your state

For Early Intervention:
Contact your municipal, county or state Deptartment of Health or
Social Services

For Services for children age 3 and up:
Contact your local board of education or state Department of Education

For financial assistance:
Contact your state Department of Health about assistance at the state
level through the federal Medical Rehabilitation Act. This act has a
different name in each state.

For other information:
Contact a medical social worker your hospital for a listing of all state
and local agencies.

INDEX